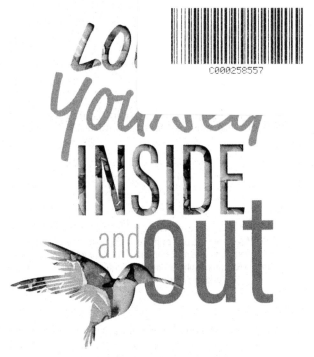

Love Yourself INSIDE and out

FAITH CANTER

EMPOWERED
BOOKS

Published in 2017 by Empowered books

Copyright © Faith Canter 2017

Fait Canter has asserted her right to be identified as the author of this
Work in accordance with the Copyright, Designs and Patents Act 1988

ISBN Paperback: 978-0-9957047-2-5
Ebook: 978-0-9957047-3-2

A CIP catalogue copy of this book can be found in the British Library.

Published with the help of Indie Authors World

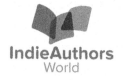

IndieAuthors
World

DEDICATION

To James,

I knew even before writing this book that it would be dedicated to you. It seems such an insignificant gesture for someone so important to my journey of being the greatest version of me I can be. Your support, encouragement, and love will always be held close to my heart.

This is for all the beautiful years we spent together as a couple, and the love-filled friendship we now share.

I will always be deeply grateful for you, for us, for our fur-babies, and for the lessons we learned together and from being apart.

With deepest love, gratitude, and respect,

Always, Faith xx

CONTENTS

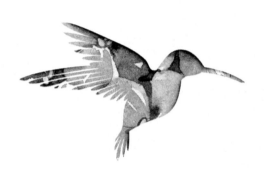

FOREWORD

L iving a heart-centred life is not the easy path, and over the years that I've known Faith, her honesty, authenticity, and integrity have always shone through. One of the many things that I love about Faith is that she lives with an open mind and heart. She isn't afraid to admit when she has made a mistake, and her mind and heart are always open enough to enable her to make the shift that she needs to make. Her ability to heal herself has enabled her to learn so much, and to clear so much, so that she can step into the life she has always wanted.

Here in her writings, she bares it all, shows her vulnerability, but also her learning. This book takes you on a journey of faith, with Faith, as she shares her learning through her experiences, and offers you the wisdom she gleaned while moving past the obstacles that were in her way. She brings the benefit of her experience into your hands, with exercises that you can get stuck into, things to think about and, most of all, a friendly voice that understands what you may be going through, too.

Nobody is perfect. We all know this intrinsically, but do we really believe it? When we live in a world where we tend to compare ourselves from the inside out to people we only see at surface level, this book gives a refreshing perspective. We rarely get the opportunity to dive deep into someone else's world and learn that we are all the same and we all have similar struggles. And it's even better to be offered a way through them, too.

Faith is beautiful on the outside and on the inside. Through her reflection, this book shows how beautiful we all are on the inside, too. And if you can catch a glimpse of your own beauty here, even for just a second, then it's most definitely worth a read.

Abby Wynne

Author of *How to Be Well*, published by Hay House

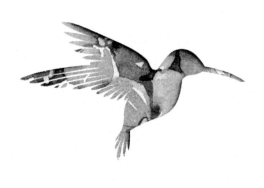

FROM THE AUTHOR

With my history of abuse, self-harm, eating disorders, and drug use, it's not really surprising that I had an obsessive hate, distrust, and disgust of everything that made me *me*. What I've found, however, is that you don't even have to go through these things to have that same level of dislike for yourself. What happens is that we accept this hate of self as normal – most other people feel it, so it must be normal, right? But this is so wrong, sooooo wrong!

What makes this worse is that economically speaking we aren't meant to like who we are or where we are in our lives, otherwise we wouldn't buy into wanting to 'better' ourselves. We wouldn't buy the new outfit, diet programme, car, house, sofa, make-up, or whatever it is that we feel will complete us or allow us to 'fit in'. Being part of our consumerist world is like buying into never being enough; it's big business, and it's what keeps many of the businesses out there going.

I admit I used to base much of my own self-worth on the way I looked, the home I kept, the relationship I was in, the job I held, and the number of friends I had. But none of that creates happiness; none of that creates fulfilment; and none of that nurtures our soul. The only thing that will ever bring us long-term love, joy, happiness, and fulfilment is knowing that we are perfectly enough, just as we are.

You see, it's an inside job. Everything we could possibly ever need to live the life of our dreams is within us!

I know you've probably heard all this before, but I'm telling you I was the queen of self-hate. I contemplated suicide more times than I can possibly count, and I pushed more people away than I care to remember. If there were prizes for this sort of thing, I would have won my fair share of them... and probably been pleased with myself for being good at something, at long last. Joking aside, I've lived far too many years of my life hating my very existence – and now? Well, now I don't.

I love and respect myself, my body, and my life. I love and respect all that brought me to the place I am in right now – all the perceived bad and horrible things in my life; all the times I allowed myself to be used and abused by others, but most importantly, by myself. I am beautiful, I am whole, and I am perfect. And I want you to feel this fully, too.

We did not come to this planet to spend a lifetime hating everything that makes us *us*! In fact, the opposite is true. We came here to live a life of love; consciously creating lives, communities, and a world that grows on love, that nurtures love, and that generates more love. In my opinion, love really is the answer to everything. If we could all learn to move away from fear and to love a little more, the world would be a very different – and happier – place.

In the following pages, I'll share with you what has assisted my client's and my own self-love embodiment, cutting through the crap, giving you the tools for your own self-love empowerment and a life that's wonderfully full. Be warned, though: you must do the work; I can't do that for you. If you want things to change, then be that change, day after day, until the change is just part of you and you it. Your future self will thank you for it... over and over again.

Lots and lots of love, Faith xx

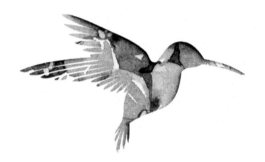

INTRODUCTION

Why is this happening to me?

As I started to write a book about loving yourself inside and out, my relationship of almost 10 years fell apart. Funny, Universe; very f-ing funny!

This man, the man I thought I would be with for the rest of my life, withdrew from me his love, comfort, support, and security, and I was left feeling betrayed, lonely, angry, and deeply, deeply hurt. I started to doubt myself again. Was I not beautiful enough? Was I not thin enough? Did I not wear the right clothes? Say the right things? Tick the right boxes? Arghhhhh, not this s#@t again! AGAIN! Really?

The thing is, I had dealt with all this 'stuff', but I was still almost totally reliant on this amazing man for my love, happiness, and fulfillment. He was my everything to me; my happiness and love was dependent on him, and not on me. It was borrowed from him, I was not generating it from within. We'd become comfortably uncomfortable in our marriage. And so, as it happens when we aren't listening to life's messages, life jolts us out of our sleepwalk with a big-ass, wake-up call.

Life was inviting me to step up, to make a change, to be more me, and to let go of my comfort blanket. Without this amazing man by my side, I had to learn to be fully me, no longer a 'we', and no longer dependent on another for what I would learn was within me (all-a-blooming-long).

I wanted to share this anonymous quote I recently read, as it explains beautifully what I am talking about: *When there is no growth, there is eventually death!*

I know that sounds harsh, but it's true. We humans need to grow (much like plants), we need to nourish and nurture ourselves otherwise growth is stunted, and things like discontent, depression, and dis-ease set in. This is true in all areas of our lives. If we don't listen to our inner knowing, eventually life shakes us up so we have no choice but to make the change we already knew we should make. If we aren't aware this is happening, we can often think that life is against us, but in fact life is working *for* us, trying to help us live the life we were meant to live. This is what happened to me with the breakdown of my marriage, and I can see clearly now it has happened repeatedly over my life to assist me in finding my way back to love, back to peace, and back to being the best version of me I can be.

People, events, places, and memories will come and go, but if we remember they are all here to assist our growth then we can pass through perceived troubles quicker, learn from them, even love the lessons we are being taught, and love the real/naked you that they are helping us to be more of. Bad things aren't happening to us just to hinder us; things are happening to wake us up, to help us grow, and to help us love more.

I know this may seem like a crazy idea when so many bad things appear to be happening to so many good people. But I am telling you, from a person that has been through her fair share of perceived crap, that becoming stuck in that place of hurt doesn't serve us or anyone else. Instead, being open to the growth these events can cause in our life and maybe considering that perhaps we have been sleepwalking through this part of our life, is one of the greatest gifts we can give ourselves.

If you don't listen to the whispers of your heart and just keep plodding on, then eventually life sends a humdinger of a message that you can no longer ignore. Then you have two choices. You either become consumed by your perceived awful life, or you accept it for what it is, then move through it and out the other side. And, guess what? Possibilities, empowerment, growth, and love await you there. They really do!

Why am I talking about all this here? In a book called *Loving Yourself Inside & Out*? Because many of the reasons we dislike ourselves is because we feel we do not 'fit in' and/or that crappy things are happening to us because we aren't a good person. But when we see that not fitting in and perceived bad things happening to us can actually be good things, it changes our focus and allows the good times to roll.

I don't believe we should just accept the crappy things we feel about ourselves, just because it's the norm or because lots of other people feel the same. I do believe, however, that by allowing our humanness, all areas of our life can blossom and grow, and we can not only realise the beauty of who we really are, but the beauty of our lives as they are.

We have everything we need within us to make this happen. We just need to relearn the concept of loving ourselves, listening to our hearts, and seeing the invitations to return to this love every time we have lost sight of it. We have everything we need within us to live a life full of love, happiness, and fulfillment.

From the breakdown of my own marriage, I found that in my aloneness, I was never alone, that a deep well of love was always within, always accessible, and always fueling me and my journey along this awesome path of life. With my husband there, I'd never attempted to access it, because I'd thought his love would be enough. But what we seek on the outside is really what we should be nurturing on the inside. An outside job is a borrowed job; an inside job is us being complete!

There have been some very dark times for me over the years, and I'm guessing there maybe have for you, too. There were times when I really didn't see the point in carrying on. But it really doesn't have to be this way. We are extraordinary beings; our body is doing millions of extraordinary things every moment of every day. Not only that, but we are travelling around on a beautiful planet in a huge and mostly undiscovered Universe, with many more billion amazing beings.

Nothing has to change for us to become happy with ourselves or our lives, other than we stop fighting ourselves and our lives. No new job, relationship, or home will do this for you; these only offer temporary, borrowed love, joy, and fulfillment. The only way to attain happiness permanently on every level is to nurture it from within. What happens then is that our outer environment follows suit, because when we move from fear to love we stop fighting ourselves – and our lives and life can't fail to follow!

Don't take my word for it. Give this book a real go, and see for yourself. Firstly, though, I'd like you to take a few deep breaths, rest your awareness in your heart, breathe in and out of your heart, and allow the energy, the breath, and the life there to expand outside of you, mixing with the rest of the world, allowing you to know you are never alone, we are all connected, and you are an embodiment of Divine Universal Love itself.

Breathe, rest, love, breathe, rest love, breathe, rest, love. You got it! Life's got you! And love's got your back!

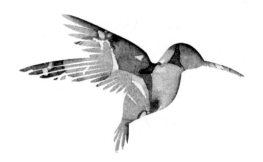

THERE'S A SELF-LOVE REVOLUTION

There's a self-love revolution going on, and you can be part of it!

There's no membership fee, funny handshakes, or weekly weigh-ins. All you need to do is let go of needing to be like everyone else. Shall I tell you why? Because everyone else is trying to be like *you*. Everyone out there (unless they are part of the revolution already) is trying to be like everyone else (who is trying to be like you). It's crazy. Everyone else thinks the next person along is the happy one. This may be because they see them as slimmer, more popular, having better hair and/or skin, nicer clothes, a more appealing personality, or that they simply just 'fit in' better.

Every day I talk with clients who are trying to 'fit in', slim-down, be loved, or find that elusive thing which will make them happy. The thing is, though, none of the other stuff you do will have long term results if you don't first embrace your love of self.

As a nutrition and detox expert, focusing on food, detoxing, and digestive health, I couldn't understand why sometimes clients would come to see me yet not stick to the healthy and healing eating plans I advised. Or if they did, they wouldn't do it long term, even though all the symptoms had gone away and they felt and looked lots better. What was going on? I'd give them all the tools for health and healing, yet they still didn't always get the desired long-term benefit.

So, I started to delve into why this was happening and, as with everything I write about, this meant looking within as well as out. It meant looking at my own journey of not only healing, but also eating disorders and body image issues.

I realized there had been big shifts in my own healing each time I'd learned to love a little more of me. Could it really be that simple? Could resolving how you feel about your body and life, allow you to heal ailments, maintain a healthy weight, and make the right life choices for yourself? Only it's not that simple, is it? Simply knowing we need to love ourselves more is completely different from actually being *able* to love ourselves. Many of us have spent a lifetime disliking everything that makes us *us*. That has then been reinforced by the media, models, marketing, and a mishmash of comments and beliefs from others about what makes a beautiful human being.

The journey to self-love is a journey of self-discovery. It's a magical, time-consuming, and empowering journey, and affects all areas of your life, not just how you feel about your body. It also affects career choices, financial freedom, your love life, and relationships with friends and family. If we are looking for a magic pill to 'fix' our lives, then embracing the love of self is life's magic pill!

If you are doing all you can for your health but getting nowhere, or you can't stick to the next new diet, programme, life change, or whatever the next new thing is that's going to 'fix' you, then maybe you should be asking yourself this instead:

How much do I really love myself and my life?

If your answer is not very much, then there's work to be done. But, luckily for you, that's where this book comes in. How do I know this? Because I've lived it. I've hated myself and my life, and I now love myself totally and unconditionally (well, most of the time – I am human, after all, but that is totally OK). This was where my own healing really started to unfold. It was also where finally, without any new fad diets, programmes or starving myself, my body weight balanced at a beautifully healthy and nourishing level. Who'd have thought that?

Think of all that time and energy that goes into hating ourselves; think of all the time wasted; all the relationships that have suffered; and all the things we haven't experienced. All because of the way we think and feel about ourselves. Think of all that time spent surviving, rather than thriving. Think of the life we can live if we could just let go of all that. How much fuller, happier, and healthier our lives could be, if we embraced our self fully and completely.

Most of the clients I work with come to me because they want to lose weight or heal a health condition. But during our sessions, we end up delving into what's behind these issues and find that when I help them discover how magical their bodies and lives are, the conditions or the extra pounds simply fade away. It is my belief that behind much of what is going on for us, are unresolved negative thoughts about ourselves and our lives. These thoughts keep us stuck in the very place we don't wish to be.

It's exhausting and disempowering to live in a state of disharmony and in a body which we dishonor and dislike. It is also – if we are honest with ourselves – completely pointless. But, what if we could use these unresolved feelings as fuel to empower a happier and healthier future? What if each one of those feelings was a key to becoming the greatest version of you that you came here to be?

When we dislike ourselves and our lives, these thoughts and feelings allow us to easily slip into the fight or flight response. This in turn causes underlying stress and anxiety, and triggers our nervous system. I call this **low level, underlying overthinking**. This hinders the body's ability to heal, makes us hold onto additional weight and toxins, and starts to break down the body's natural healthy, healing responses and reactions to all sort of daily situations, hindering its ability to uptake nutrients, digest foods, fight off infections, recall conversations, and interfering with all manner of day-to-day activities.

There is also a direct impact on our health at a cellular level; repetitively thinking these thoughts starts to reinforce these negative pathways in the brain, making it easier each time to slip into them again, and again, and again. It's a bit like when we see a clear pathway cutting through a forest, where lots of people have passed before. It's easy to find that path, stay on the path, and reinforce the path for the walkers who come behind us. If we keep following our negative thoughts, we'll keep reinforcing this pathway and find it harder and harder to find the positive path, as that starts to become overgrown and more difficult to see.

And what's worse, thinking the same thoughts over and over again makes those parts of the brain stronger, making the associated part of the body stronger/fatter/thinner/weaker, depending on our individual thoughts about them. For instance, there has been research to show that when participants just imagined playing the piano (they didn't actually do it, they just imagined it every day for a set period of time), after several weeks that part of the brain believed to be associated with playing the piano was more lit up. But that isn't the best bit. What's really impressive is that these same (non-piano playing) people's finger muscles were noticeably stronger and more pronounced, as though they had actually been playing the piano all that time.

So, if we constantly think how we hate our big belly, pointed nose, or arm fat, then our thoughts will be creating an environment within the body which reinforces the very part of our body we dislike. Ouch, that sucks, doesn't it? However, when we start loving and respecting our bodies and lives, we begin to reinforce these positive pathways (making it easier to find them each time); we reinforce these parts of the brain and body with messages of what we do want, rather than don't want; and we go from the fight or flight response to the nourish and flourish response. And that's always a much nicer place to hang out!

Just thinking happy thoughts is not enough, though; it's much more than that. But we'll cover this later in the book.

When resolving the crappy stuff which we are thinking about ourselves, we make space for new, amazing, and totally awesome stuff to unfold in our lives. We become open to seeing and embracing new possibilities which we may have been shut down to before. We have more energy for new possibilities, and we harness the power of love rather than the disempowered path of fear and loathing.

I started playing with this concept with my clients, and noticed big shifts in what was happening for them. Not only could they now embrace new healthy choices for themselves, but they enjoyed them, stuck to them, and found that these changes simply became part of their new healthy lives, rather than feeling like another 'limiting diet or programme'. This, of course, then led to more instances of healing, healthy weight goals being achieved, and people living happy, fulfilling, and harmonious lives.

And the magic doesn't stop there! I have noticed that many of my clients have then gone on to change careers, relationships, homes, and even countries, because they now understand that they are not only worthy of more, but want to embrace the life they have been gifted.

I hope you can see now how incredibly powerful this 'self-love stuff' really is. Because, without embracing the love of self, all that wonderful magical stuff you are doing physically may only be short-lived. But when we start loving, accepting, and nurturing what is, that's when the mind and body rest in a state of harmonious healing, of accepting nourishment, and of reinforcing the greatest and best of who we came here to be.

With my nutrition and detox background, it was hard for me to admit – initially – that there might actually be something much more important to harnessing health and happiness than the physical stuff. But I have seen time and time again that this is the case. No matter if it is someone trying to recover from ME/CFS, wanting to lose weight, or to have better skin. If we don't resolve what's going on underneath these disharmony 'symptoms', then the physical stuff often simply does not stick. Yet, when we resolve to love ourselves more and follow the messages to do so, the physical symptoms often fade away. And not only that, but we enjoy being who we came here to be, even more.

When we love and accept what is, that's when things change! We cannot change from a place of conflict; it must be done from a place of compassionate love instead. This is the same for all relationships, but never more important than with the relationship we have with our self.

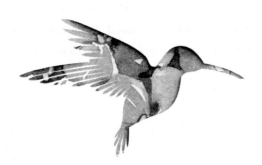

CONSCIOUSLY CREATING CHANGE

Originally, this chapter was at the end of this book, as I had thought it would be a good way to condense what had resonated with you throughout the book into a plan of action to consciously create the change you want in your life. Then I realised that if I gave you the information on how to consciously create change now, you could be doing just that whilst reading through the rest of the book.

So, whatever resonates with you during the following pages, I urge you to consciously create the change you want with it, right from the time you read it. DO NOT wait; don't put it off; don't decide you'll do it next week, after the holidays, the birthday, or the next big event. There will always be something, somewhere going on that can distract you from consciously creating the change you want. So, start now!

You have no idea how many people I work with who already know how to look after themselves mentally, physically and/or spiritually, but are not doing it. This is basically where this chapter came from. Those beautiful clients who have not implemented all they know into the change they desire.

Why is this? Why is it that we have the information on how to create the change we want, yet don't do it? Well, there are two reasons. One is that we lack the love of self to make the nourishing and nurturing choices for ourselves (which is basically what this book is all about). The second reason is that we lack a conscious plan of action. We leave the workshop, course, training, programme, book, article, video or webinar, all fired up, all ready to 'make that change'. But then we get home, life gets in the way, and we forget about it until we attend the next workshop, read the next book, etc. And generally, the process starts again.

Sometimes we do implement some running, introduce green smoothies, going to bed early, meditating, etc. Often, these changes last a few days, sometimes a few weeks, or if it's a health mission it sometimes stays a lot longer than that. I usually find that if people are in a really bad way mentally or physically, they find it easier to stick to things long term, because they basically feel so bloody awful they give anything a go. This is life forcing us to make the change that we've probably been thinking about for ages. Our body and mind have been whispering to us for soooo long that eventually they shout and we feel so bad we'll try and usually stick to anything. What happens more often than not, though, is we keep doing the good things until we feel better, and then bit by bit these practices slowly drop off. Then a year or five later, we suddenly wonder why we don't feel so tip-top any more. I've been there, too. I know this is what we often do to ourselves, then sit there wondering why this is happening again.

Let me give you an example. As I got well from ME/CFS and started doing more things, sometimes I would 'forget' to meditate a couple of times a day, or use Tapping/Emotional Freedom Technique (EFT) on what was coming up for me, or to eat really nourishing food in a nurturing way. I would then slowly start to dip and wonder why, because I had thought I had recovered. I couldn't understand what had gone wrong, and then I would realise I wasn't fueling my mind, body, and soul in the right way.

Some people said to me, 'If you still have to do these "healthy" things for yourself, then you have not recovered!" What rubbish! To live in the modern world, everyone should be fueling themselves in the right way to prevent feeling depleted by life's demands. Anyway, I digress. What I am trying to explain is that, when we make sure that every day – in as many ways as possible – we are fueling the life we want to lead with the fuel that is going to encourage this empowerment, then we will find that we get back what we desire from our mind, body, and soul. So, to fuel ourselves in the right way, we need to consciously create a daily practice that does just that.

How do we do that? We create a conscious plan of action. And by this, I don't mean a vague or perhaps rough plan in our heads, where we tell our self 'tomorrow I will go to the gym, have a green smoothie for breakfast, and meditate'. I am guessing that you may have already tried this approach before? To create a conscious action plan, we need to get the vagueness out of our heads, onto paper, into our computer, or on our phone.

If you're anything like me, then this 'brain dump' of ideas firstly frees up that pesky mind for more nourishing and nurturing things, and secondly allows you to see what you are going to do when, what are going to be your non-negotiables, and what timescale you have to do them in. Eventually, the plan will become a new healthy habit, but until then, let's make that plan happen!

As you work your way through this book, really feel what resonates for you, or if some of the contents remind you of other things you once did or thought about doing but did not actually follow through with. When this happens, commit to consciously adding these things into your daily routine, even if only for a few moments a day (if that's all you think you can manage at the moment). Then get out your diary, calendar, journal, phone, computer, whatever it takes, and start scheduling these things into your day/week. Right there and then, as these ideas resonate with you! Not later, when you have finished the book, or whenever you have more time, or when you remember to do so. Start scheduling them in right then and there. Better still, stop reading and *do* them, then and there. For example, if it's meditation, put the book down and take a quick 10 minutes' meditation time. I can guarantee you that if you take 10 minutes to do what resonates with you in that moment, you will feel more inspired and empowered to schedule that into your day moving forward.

For me, my day starts with me getting up around 5am (in the summer) and 6am in the winter. I work best in the mornings; I'm usually in the zone then for doing things, and have the energy to do them. I love that quiet time of the day before the rest of the world wakes up. I get up and meditate straight away (otherwise, life can get in the way and it's dinner time and I may not have meditated). I then do roughly an hour of yoga, and then sometimes I journey (a Shamanic practice that I love), then I walk the dogs in the woods (with my heart wide open – more about this later on), come home and have a green smoothie, juice or a cup of herbal tea, and a soak in the bath with a good book.

I usually start seeing clients from about 10am. If I am feeling tired, drained, or uninspired during the day, I see this as an invitation to make some more 'me time' and meditate, journey, read, or go for a walk. I am then able to function at the higher level I like, and serve my clients to the best of my ability. I eat good food in a really nourishing way and drink plenty of fluids, and I stop work about 4pm usually. Sometimes I work in the evenings, but mainly on small admin tasks while I watch inspiring movies and documentaries which lift my spirit and nurture my soul.

I go to bed early, because this is what my body and mind prefer, and I meditate, journal, and sometimes journey before I do so. Throughout my week, I schedule in walking time, as this connection with myself and nature is something that really fills me up and makes me feel alive. I also schedule in plenty of 'me time'. Sundays I call 'self-love Sunday', because I don't work, see friends, or plan anything. This is my day to recharge, plan, and nourish. If all of these things do not go into my schedule, I know from past experience that my week fills up with other things, and I end up feeling depleted and uninspired because I am not filling my cup from the inside out. What can also happen is that three hours after logging onto Facebook, etc, I find I have done nothing, feel fed-up, and have wasted three hours of my life.

I realise that not everyone has such a flexible schedule, but you can still consciously create change in what time you do have. Be honest with yourself: how much of your time is wasted on Facebook, TV, or just feeling tired (because you are not fueling yourself correctly)? Could you borrow back some of this time? Maybe not all of it, but perhaps half, or even a quarter of it?

I know that the more I meditate, the less sleep I need. Also, I am more creative, inspired, aligned, and productive when I meditate regularly. When I was writing my second book, *Cleanse – The Holistic Detox Program for Mind, Body and Soul,* I was meditating seven or eight times a day/night and I flew through the book with hardly any sleep for about six weeks. The thing is, though, I felt amazing. I was on fire, and in the zone! You may not feel as though you have time right now to consciously create the change you desire, but when you are fueling yourself with things like meditation and thinking and eating better, you generate more time by default – and you will be more productive in that time.

When we start setting aside time for nourishing things which we may not consider necessary in our life, we will find that 'doing less' amounts to achieving more. Trust me, I have seen this time and time again. **If we wish to achieve more in our life, we need to nourish and nurture more!** Not, push more, be more or do more... that, in fact, depletes our 'achieving' reserves.

One of the super simple things I have many of my clients do is to set reminders/alarms in their phone or computer calendars which go off either every hour or every two hours. These are to remind them to drop into their hearts, be present, accept where they are, or Tap/EFT on the last negative thought they just had. These reminders have produced amazing results. No matter what they are doing at that time, they stop for just 10-30 seconds and connect with the things they are consciously trying to create in their life. These reminders soon become habits, and their way of thinking throughout the day soon changes to a much more positive way of being. They have consciously created the change they wanted with just a few simple reminders (things don't have to be difficult or complicated; quite the opposite, in fact).

Remember when consciously creating change, to value your you-time. And not only that, but value your time, full-stop! Don't spread yourself too thin, making time for everyone and everything else and neglecting to spend time on you. You cannot look after others long-term if you don't look after yourself first. Plus, you'll make the people around you much happier when you're happy, too!

In my workshops, I often ask attendees if they would make the changes they desired if it was for someone else they loved – and always, they answer yes. This allows them to see how they would find a way to make these things happen if they loved themselves as much as they loved others. So, I ask you the same: if you had to make these changes in your life for a loved one, would you find a way?

I know change can be frightening. I have my spent my life afraid of change on one hand, and desperate for things to change on the other. Sometimes it feels easier to hold onto what we know rather than let go and move into what we don't know, even if the 'what we know' isn't making us happy any more. How many relationships, jobs, friends, habits, belongings, or homes have we held onto because it was familiar and sometimes easy, but did not fill us up any more? Honestly, ask yourself this: how much of your own power, energy, vitality, life have you given away by staying 'comfortable', but often unhappy.

If you keep walking that 'comfortable' path and aren't moving towards a life you love which fills you up and nourishes and nurtures your soul, then life will make this change happen for you. It's like the blueprint of the world. Despite what we are programmed to think, we humans did not come to this planet to 'make do'; we came here to live, to love, and to connect. And when we continue to live lives that are not in keeping with these higher versions of ourselves, then life likes to help us along towards our real reason for being here. It's a real case of making do just won't do!

Allowing yourself to step beyond your comfort zone will never serve you wrong. You'll feel growth, expansion, connection, clarity, and a new-found strength and power in the uncomfortable. So, make sure some of your conscious creation is about stepping beyond where you are now; that's how the change you desire actually happens, when you step beyond what you already know.

Consciously creating change not only applies to health and well-being goals, but to future long-term goals. Quite often when I am working with clients who have been ill for some time, we also try to figure out what it is they want from their life (long term) and how they can start moving towards this goal (if only one baby step at a time). Why do I do this with people who have been poorly for so long? Because usually they are struggling to see a future for themselves, and that's not a healthy place to be in. So, rather than focusing on the way things were once in the past, or trying to get back their previous health, relationships, or life, we instead focus on creating a full, healthy, and loving future for them, using what they have learned – previously and because of their illness – as their fuel for their empowerment.

I find that time and time again, once they start picturing and moving towards a life of their dreams, they also start to make progress with their health. Because the 'stuckness' starts to finally shift. Even if the conscious change they create is simply signing up for a free online programme in a topic that interests them, or reading a few books about the subject, or watching one YouTube video a day. They start to feel their way into this reality and start believing it for themselves. When we become stationary in our lives and are not growing in some way, we can start to feel a little stuck or even dead inside. We need to feel growth as human beings; we are much the same as plants in this way. If we do not feel like we are growing as a person then how can we consciously create growth?

=What can we do regularly to move towards our long-term goals? Even if it's just reading one page of a book on the topic a day – we can all do that, right? Or listen to podcasts in the car, rather than the radio? Whatever you can do, schedule it in, consciously create the change, until it becomes a new and beautiful habit and you feel you are growing, evolving, and moving towards your goals.

Here's the serious bit...

Things will not change unless you consciously create the change!

Or they will change, but you won't like the way life decides to change things for you, because it will most likely be a big-ass-wake-up-call instead. I am all for the Law of Attraction stuff, but you still have to get up, show up, and wake up, otherwise life will wake *you* up!

So, please don't just read this book cover to cover and not use what resonated with you to create the life you desire. Consciously create the change you desire in each of your days, and things *will* change.

> *Your job is to open doors. Their job is to decide whether they have the courage to walk through them.*
> ### – *Solomon*

(From *Solomon Speaks* – Dr Eric Pearl & Frederick Ponzlow)

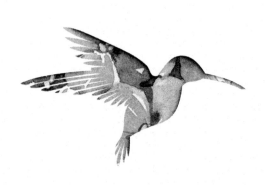

SELF-LOVE SURVIVAL GUIDE

Consciously creating change is also about recognising when something isn't working, and knowing how to consciously change it into something that is.

In my last book, *Cleanse – A Holistic Detox Program for Mind, Body & Soul,* I talked about my Feeling Blue List. It's such an easy thing to do, and has assisted lots of people I've worked with to understand when they have lost their way and how to find their route back. The Self-Love Survival Guide is my new improved version of the Feeling Blue List, with a new, softer, and more positive name! YAY!

We know that when we are in a bad headspace we will convince ourselves that we have tried everything within our power to change it. That we have been eating well, meditating, being grateful, and a whole heap of other things. But, in fact, if we were honest with ourselves and not trying to play mind games, we probably haven't. We may have sat down to meditate, but ended up simply listing all the crappy things happening at that moment.

It's so easy for things to slip and we don't realise why. When we are feeling good, we often forget to do all the things we know help us both mentally and physically. And then, when we are not feeling so good, stuff starts to build up and we are less prepared for it. Before we know it, we are totally consumed by the negativity of whatever is happening to us. Yet, every time without fail, we convince ourselves that we have done everything we should/could be doing to resolve this situation.

One day after I had been feeling pretty crappy again, I asked myself what I could do to break this habit, and it suddenly dawned on me creating something as simple as a short list was what I could do. So, I did it!

My list has evolved over the time I have been using it, and I have a version saved to my laptop and on my phone, so that I always have easy access to it in times of need. And, I'm telling you, it really, really works!

So, what you need to do (in a good frame of mind) to create such a list, is to get a piece of A4 paper and draw two lines down it, to create three columns. At the top of the first column, write 'What Nurtures'; at the top of the middle one, write 'Naughty Notes'; and at the top of the last one, write 'Conscious Change'.

> In the first column, write a list of all the things you know assist your health, happiness, and harmony. These may be things you have tried in the past, or simple things like taking a bath, meditating, getting out in nature, or they may be some of the things from this book which resonate with you.

> In the second column, consider ways in which you can get through to your not-so-emotionally-strong self that you may not be doing the things on the list. Put the list in order of things that work for you, and then you can work your way down as and when you need to.

➢ In the last column, write down how you are going to consciously make sure these things start to happen for your health, happiness, and harmony.

You will notice from my list that I wrote meditating down, and then next to it I have asked myself if I am REALLY meditating, or am I just trying to convince myself I am when really I've been sitting listing everything that's rubbish right now or making a shopping list in my head. You need to be honest with yourself, and you need to keep updating and referring to the list as and when you need to. It's surprising how many wonderful things we stop doing for ourselves, simply because we get out of the habit of it.

Here's my current Self-Love Survival Guide to give you an idea of how to fill out your own:

Self-Love Survival Guide		
What Nurtures?	**Naughty Notes**	**Conscious Change**
Are you Meditating?	Really?	Meditate for 20mins every morning
	From a place of nourishment, or from a place of trying to fix, change or improve?	Do a 3 min meditation at lunch
	Perhaps you need to change your meditation?	Meditate when I cannot sleep at night
	Have you convinced yourself this doesn't work, when you know it does, Faith?	
You know you're enough, don't you, Faith?	If you don't, then use this as an invitation to resolve that feeling & return to your heart	Feel into these feelings right now, and see what they are inviting you to be more of

Self-Love Survival Guide

What Nurtures?	Naughty Notes	Conscious Change
You know this is happening for you, Faith?	It's a redirection not a rejection	What's the gift here?
Are you listening to your body?	Really?	What is your body telling you?
	Or are you just creating a list of ailments?	Where's your thinking gone?
	Are you seeing the ailments as invitations to resolve an imbalance?	What is your body inviting you to become in harmony with?
Have you tried accepting this?	Accepting allows you to let go of the conflict	If you cannot change it, can you accept it?
Are you caught up in the story?	It's often your thinking that is the problem, not the actual problem any more	Let the story/the thinking go then
Where are you hanging out at the moment?	Head or heart?	Set reminders to hang out in heart more, and do more heart-centred meditations
Are you willing to experience everything?	Or are you trying to fix, change, or improve?	Feel all the feelings, even the perceived bad, then you'll feel the good even more
	Conflict causes dis-ease, you know, Faith!!	
Have you tried letting go of this?	Ask yourself: can I let go of this now?	Breathe and let it go!
Are you tapping?	On what you are already internalizing, or on what you think is wrong?	Tap on the raw emotions, Faith, unedited!

Self-Love Survival Guide		
What Nurtures?	**Naughty Notes**	**Conscious Change**
	Go on, you know it works!	
Are you listening to upbeat music daily?	Or is it the same old songs on the radio?	Listen to happy music when getting ready each morning
	Are the songs slightly depressive?	
Are you watching and reading inspiring/ empowering stuff?	Have an inspiring movie day!	Watch at least two inspiring things a week
Have you taken yourself on a mini adventure recently?	Why not? You know you love them and they nurture you	Go on one right now, and schedule in three a week from now on
		Now, consciously create the change, by scheduling this in!

I have found, time and time again, that no matter how determined and inspired we are, unless we get our thoughts, plans, and actions out of our heads and onto paper, things often don't happen. So, let's start with the Self-Love Survival Guide so that it allows us to be in a better frame of mind for the rest.

On the following page is a template of the Self-Love Survival Guide for you to use. Copy it, print it out, fill it in, and save it wherever you feel would best benefit you when you are feeling a little low.

Self-Love Survival Guide		
What Nurtures?	**Naughty Notes**	**Conscious Change**
		Now consciously create the change, by scheduling this in!

Here, I wanted to add a little bit about slowing down. Yes, it's good to consciously create change and to create your Self-Love Survival Guide, but remember to add 'down-time' to both of these. Everything on the planet needs a reboot occasionally. Technology does, obviously, but humans do just as much. If you do not put aside 'rebooting' time, then life will add it in for you. This could be in the form of a bad headache, a cold, or a bad back. Have you ever noticed that all of those ailments or problems come at the most inconvenient times, when you simply don't have the time for them? But they are usually so debilitating that you have no choice but to take some time out and reboot. So, why not schedule this time in yourself, before life does it for you?

It's in the down-time that we get inspiration, find our way around obstacles, recharge, re-energize, and indeed reboot. It's when we also stop long enough to take our 'busy blinkers' off and notice the pure joy, beauty, and life around us that we often don't notice as we go about our day-to-day lives. Life is magical, beautiful, and expansive, when we allow ourselves to view it with a heart wide open, and this is more easily done when we slow life down a little.

When we slow down, sometimes way down, that's when we rise up and see the beauty that is all around us, the beauty that is always around us. And if we slow down even more, then we start to see the beauty that is in us – the preciousness, worth and value that was there all along.

Lori Cash Richards,

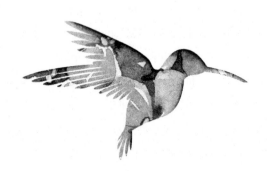

CONSCIOUSLY AWARE

Today, give yourself permission to break free of any old habits, beliefs, and programming which hold you in a state of unconscious living. Surrender to what this day will bring, and wake up to conscious, fulfilling living. Do you give yourself permission? Breathe into it now, and soften around it; allow the permission to filter through and the resistances to slowly dissolve.

Generally, we are wandering through life distracted, not being consciously aware, not noticing what's right in front of us, sleepwalking, until something wakes us up, even if only for a moment. Have you ever noticed you can drive to work, the shops, or school, and have no idea how you got there? You were asleep! Have you ever noticed you get up, make a cuppa, have a shower, dress, and walk out the door, but have no real memories of this? You were asleep! Have you ever noticed you can sit through a whole film or TV programme and not be able to recall most of it? You were asleep! The list goes on and on.

We spend much of our day distracted by our thoughts, by our habits, programmes, and memories. Occasionally, though, something wakes us up. But to do this, it needs to be something intense. It could be an accident, a big surprise, a fright, a loss, a gain, or it could be a stunning view or a magical evening of some kind. These memories – good or bad – are then stuck in our mind, because they woke us up from sleepwalking. Even what we perceive to be bad things are actually good, as they are showing us life in all its technicoloured glory – we are no longer distracted, but instead interacting with life. The other good thing is that we can practise the art of being consciously aware of ourselves, of life and the planet, from a space of open-hearted awareness. And the more we practise and nurture this new habit, the easier it is to be in this place moving forward.

But what is being in open-hearted awareness? Being aware means you become aware of your thoughts and actions, but more as a spectator than being pulled under and into the story of why they are there/happening. It's much the same as meditation; you become aware of the thoughts but not consumed by them. With awareness of our thoughts, we can become aware of the craziness of our brain, but we don't get stuck in it. We can step away, see our craziness, own it, and let it go much more easily. When I refer to open-hearted awareness, what I am talking about is viewing what's going on with an open heart, rather than a judgmental head. This allows us to not only become aware of our thoughts and actions, but to be open and loving to them and also to our fellow human beings' thoughts and actions. When we see the world through love rather than fear, the world itself appears to change. But what has mostly happened is that we have just changed the way we view ourselves, each other, and the world as a whole.

I wrote this poem about the power of awareness, and I wanted to share it with you here because I know it sounds too simple to be effective. But, in my opinion, simple always wins over that compli-cated, crazy brain, any day...

I've read books, books with beautiful words and magical beings, just like you, but not like me.

They were inspiring, empowering even, but clearly not true, or perhaps I was less deserving, less spiritual, lacking, not enough to even be enough, to feel enough, to be worthy of those words working for me.

Sometimes I'd feel a little better for a little while, I'd feel whoopy, I've got it, I'm fixed, I'm happy... oh crap, no I'm not!

This was the cycle, this made for more doubt, it's exhausting searching for what others have but that you are without.

Always searching, always hoping, never quite achieving and so the cycle goes on.

Could it be so simple, could it be so easy? Surely not, this must be wrong.

No, it really works, this simple technique, I feel it, I am it, but how?

How can a lifetime of troubles be so easily sorted by something so simple as being open-heartedly aware of my thoughts and actions in my current incarnation on this big ball of gas, that we call Earth?

Why am I talking about awareness of thoughts and actions, when it comes to loving yourself and your life more? Because it's the stories of how we feel things should be, haven't been, need to be, or how we feel others treat us, or how we treated others, that keeps us stuck in the not loving, not feeling worthy, and not feel-ing good enough. When we realise that they really are all stories and – for the most part – not real, then we can let them go and become aware of the magic of our existence, of our community, and of this planet instead.

As one of my favorite authors, Anthony de Mello, says: *It's time to wake-up!* And, with our waking up comes the awareness of the beauty of who we are, and why we are here. Let's all wake up!

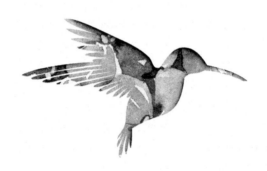

ACCEPTANCE

It is because I love you that I don't engage in the drama of your perceived problems. Today I see the best in you so that you can too!

Sandy C Newbigging

For years, the idea of acceptance puzzled me. Actually, it more than puzzled me; I couldn't get my head around it at all. In fact, it frightened the bejesus out of me. How could I accept this crap was my life and would be my life forever? Nooooooo!

What I didn't realise was that when we accept where we are in life, our health conditions, our body image, relationships, etc, we are then able to move forward with much more ease and grace towards the best version of us we came here to be.

We are so attached to the outcome all the time. We say things to our self like: I'll be happy when I am thin, on holiday, in my new house, relationship, or career. We are so attached to outcomes, to future happiness that we aren't present in the... well, in the present. We become so fixated on the way something should turn out that we close down to any other possibilities. We don't see life's gifts and magnificence, and we often think life is against us when nothing could be further from the truth.

Years ago, I used to say, 'If I don't expect anything, then I'm never disappointed.' This was because I felt like I was continuously being let down. Although my sentiment was way off, the words were actually fairly accurate. Resolve the attachment to your expectation(s) and you'll never be disappointed. Not because you'll be right about being let down, but because things will start happening that you never thought were possible without you even getting involved. The attachment to an outcome causes conflict, and closes you off to seeing new and amazing possibilities and the beauty of life unfolding for your greater good. When you let go of how you think something should be, whatever is *actually* meant to be can unfold.

When you feel yourself getting upset about a health condition, relationship, body image, or in fact anything in life, you have gone into that low-level, underlying, overthinking that I talked about previously. You'll then start reinforcing that very thing you don't want in your life within your brain and nervous system. So, instead, why not try acceptance? Trust me, this stuff works!

Simply trying not to feel a certain way, distracting yourself from your thoughts, thinking positive thoughts or just saying affirmations, doesn't work for most people. This is because if you don't believe what you are saying and/or thinking, then you will again go into low-level, underlying, overthinking, because you will be in conflict with what you are saying to yourself. You cannot be in conflict with something and move forward from it; it just doesn't work that way, I'm afraid. Neither can you ignore your 'problems' away, or distract yourself to health. Those pesky thoughts are still there at a subconscious level, triggering all sorts of unhelpful responses to all sorts of day-to-day things. Plus, they will never just magically go away of their own accord; they'll just fester underneath.

So, how do you accept the unacceptable?

When you notice that you have been triggered by something – it might be 30 seconds, 30 minutes, or 30 hours later – you simply rest into it. You allow that feeling to be there, rather than getting carried away by the story of how it came to be there. You can say to yourself things like:

It's ok to feel this way.

I'm human and this is a normal human response.

It's ok to be upset, angry, tired, peed-off, jealous, disappointed, etc.

I'm ok with feeling this way right now.

I'm ok with this right now.

I'm not going to fight this right now.

I'm not going to fight myself right now.

I'm consciously letting go of this reaction right now.

I surrender to whatever this is or whatever is going on.

I surrender to the fact this is happening for my greater good.

I'm letting go of my need for this to be anything other than what it is right now.

Find a phrase that works for you in the moment, one that allows you to accept yourself and/or your life as it is right now. Personally, I find that when I am triggered by something, I soften (breathing, opening, and allowing) into the feeling, which allows it to flow. So, if someone says something to me and it triggers a negative response/feeling/memory in me, then I feel myself physically and mentally soften into it, embracing it and my human reaction to the situation. Then it feels like I am just going with the flow, instead of trying to swim against the current of my own emotional conflict. We all know how hard that is, though, right?

Author Eckhart Tolle say that it's never the problem that is the problem, but our way of thinking about the problem that is. This is so true. You can choose a different reality to the one you have slipped into. You can choose to soften into your perceived problem, and thus go with the flow of life instead. I am constantly surprised how quickly (in fact, instantly) that this habit of acceptance turns something which I would have perceived as really stressful into something beautiful. There's a learning in everything, and with acceptance you leave yourself open to that learning, and to flowing right through whatever it was that you perceived to be your problem. So, next time you find yourself in conflict, try to soften and flow into it; maybe say one of the above list (if one resonates with you); and accept where you are right now and your humanness. In doing so, you make room for a much fuller and less conflicted life to unfold.

Feel the feelings to let them flow!

Remember that most of the time busyness is just a distraction; a distraction from our thoughts, feelings, emotions, soul's calling, all of these and more. We need to feel, we need to listen in, and we need to slow down, to learn how to be more of what we came here to be.

I was recently emailing my ex-husband, and I said in the email, 'Who'd have thought I would have found my happy on the flipside of all those feelings I spent a lifetime trying not to feel?' You see, when we keep trying not to feel the 'bad stuff', it makes it even harder to feel the good stuff, too! That's another beautiful reason to accept where we are, feel how we feel, and let those feelings flow.

With all the awful things happening in the world, I know it can feel hard to accept life. The thing is, when we realise that all these events are here to help us grow both individually and together as the human race, then they don't seem so awful after all.

I recently had a client come to see me who was having issues with their boss at work. They said they understood that everything happens for a reason and that everything happens to help us/them grow, but said this could not be the case with their boss because everyone in their department was feeling the same way. So, how on earth could they all need the same lessons and learnings at the same time? My reply was that if everyone was feeling the same way then that meant everyone in the department could be part of a bigger change that was required; they could all have slipped from love, and were all being invited to slip back into it. And that is what we are all being invited to do all the time – to return to love. The problem is that most of us are unaware that this is what we are being invited to do; we think the world is against us. But it's not! It's inviting us to make a change, be the change, invite more change from more people, and to stop fighting ourselves, each other, and life.

Life isn't against you, dear reader. Life is inviting you to be the best of you which you can be! I know that sounds a bit backwards when crappy things happen, but those crappy things happen because we are fighting ourselves, each other, and life. We aren't loving; we're living in fear instead! But, when we practise acceptance (let's face it, the opposite doesn't get us anywhere, anyway), we move away from fear and conflict with ourselves and everything around us, and move into flow, into ease, and into a life of love, fulfillment, and happiness.

Practising acceptance saved me from myself when my marriage came to an end. The old, non-accepting, non-loving, life-hating Faith would have fallen into a pit of despair and believed myself and the world to be all the worse for it. I would have blamed him, me, those around me, and life, for serving up another plate of suck-ass. And that would have allowed me to live on depression street for all the longer.

This time, though, things were different, I was different, and I knew that old pattern didn't serve me. Instead, I knew I would grow, live, and love all the more from this experience if I could learn to accept that it was here to help me return to love. So, I accepted it. It wasn't always easy and I fell off the wagon here and there, but I embraced and accepted that part of me as well. I was no longer going to give myself a hard time for being me, for being human. None of this 'I should know better' crap, just love for myself, for him, and for where we both were in our lives.

The gratitude that came through for him, for our life together, and for the future we would both have for sharing the best part of 10 years together, flooded through and out of me. We grew more in those months of separating than we had together in a very long time. The love, compassion, and understanding we shared in those months touched us both deeply. I was yet again reminded that everything, every single thing in life, is happening to open us up to love. Even in losing someone you deeply love, you can find more love than you had ever imagined before.

Know as I am writing this that my life is filled with more love than I ever felt was possible. I get love from every direction every day. It's the most incredible feeling to feel so much love in my life and in the world.

Practising acceptance allows us to soften and flow into life's challenges, seeing life's possibilities and returning to life's loves.

So much energy is wasted on fighting ourselves, each other, and life. It's completely pointless. It does not serve us, and instead diminishes our resources at every level. I am not saying you must let it slide when someone does something crappy, what I am saying is it does nothing to fight them and your feelings about them. Accepting that it has happened and what they did, allows you to move through it quicker than harbouring negative feelings, emotions, and stresses about them. You'll then return to that place of love quicker and more easily see life's opportunities open up from this perceived wrong.

Every single perceived crappy thing in my life led me to a more wondrous and fulfilling point in my life. Every single time! Once I accepted my abuse as a child, I learned how much stronger a person it has made me, and how it is possible to truly love anyone. When I accepted the people I'd allowed to use and abuse me, I realised how damaging self-hate really is and there became no other option than to love myself and them fully. When I accepted my years of being housebound with ME/CFS, I realised it was one of my greatest gifts of all; it saved my life, as it gave me no other choice than to make some big changes in my life. Before my husband and I found each other, I was in a relationship with what most people describe as an evil man. But, with acceptance of that relationship and what he unknowingly taught me, I feel a deep understanding and strength within me. And, as I explained above, when my marriage broke down I found more love in my life than I had experienced in the whole of my life put together. And do you know where it came from? Within; it came from within! When I look back, all the health ailments, people, places, and events have given me great gifts and allowed me to discover greater depths of me. If I'd known and understood the power of acceptance back then, I wonder where I would be now. Even so, the power of accepting all that came before has supercharged my life to a whole new level of love, ease, and flow. Perceived bad things still happen, but I know they are redirections so I work with acceptance to allow them to flow, and I fight myself and my life a little less each time.

Our fears, doubts, discomforts, and disillusionments can all be fuel to a fulfilling life. In the process of acceptance, we fall into a place of listening for life's whispers. We stop fighting, and start embracing life instead. We find our strength, abundance, life's beauty becomes supercharged, and the love flows with more ease into our life. Why? Because we have let down our walls, eased through our barriers, and opened our heart to life's possibilities. When we are not in a place of acceptance, we can be closed off to much of this so it becomes much harder to see life's magic and thus to embrace and love it.

But how do we accept our bodies, when many of us dislike them so much?

There was no way on this planet I was going to accept my body. I hated the way it looked. The only time I had even remotely liked it was when I was super-thin, due to eating disorders and/or drug use. And then, because of the eating disorder and/or drug use, I didn't love it because I couldn't love me.

To top it off, not only was I bigger than I wanted to be (even though I ate all the right foods), but I believed myself to be ugly, and there were various other things about my body which I disliked with a passion. Acceptance of my body was not an option! But part of me knew that when we are thinking about something so often and so passionately, we are actually reinforcing those pathways in the brain and thus reinforcing the very things we don't like. Not accepting our bodies reinforces the very things we do not like.

I started to accept my body, by acknowledging all the wonderful things that it was doing for me and which made it easier to accept. Sure, it hadn't always been healthy, but it still got me from A-B, it was pumping blood around it every second of every day, and also doing a million other, different, automatic responses which I wasn't even aware of. It's actually a miracle how many wonderful things the body is doing all the time without us even realising it. We are walking, blinking miracles, that's what we are!

I then started to pick out things on my body that I like – my eyes, bum, and legs – and really started to not only accept but appreciate these things when I looked in the mirror. I also realised that although as a child I had hated my freckles, I really didn't hate them now. Bit by bit I accepted more and more of my body, creating mini body gratitude lists every day when in the shower, getting dressed, or standing in front of the mirror. I started praising more and more of my body inside and out. Even the dreaded belly started to receive my love and appreciation (although perhaps not acceptance to start with, ha!). I began to realise that even it was doing many amazing things every day. I massaged it, loved it, and thanked it for being part of me. When I had crappy thoughts about this or any other part of my body, I would remind myself it's ok to be human, it's ok to have these thoughts, but that I was no longer going to base my beauty on them.

Shockingly, my weight started to stabilise and I began to see the real beauty in myself. This in turn created greater confidence. Someone recently said to me that confidence is far more attractive than any 'made-up' person (someone who spends a lot of time and energy looking good). You see, true beauty – as with true happiness, joy, and love – comes from within. When we are confident, people are attracted to that, they want to be around us, they want to be with us. How the heck did I never understand this all those years ago? I spent a lifetime hating myself and putting myself down, only to realise that this was exactly the thing making me unattractive (in my mind) to others.

Acceptance on all levels is what allows us to live a full, happy, healthy, and loving life. So, when we notice our thoughts have slipped into a negative way of thinking about our self, our life, or someone or something else, be ok with our humanness. Be ok with the thoughts, and then be ok with whatever the thoughts are about. We are quite obsessed these days with 'thinking positive' and being 'light-workers', etc, but we can only be the fullest and greatest versions of ourselves if we embrace the shadow side of us. This means embracing, accepting, and then learning to love all parts of us, especially the parts we dislike – our unwanted shadow side. When you love that side, too, you will feel true freedom, true growth, and true love in yourself and your life.

Meditating is another way I rest into the acceptance of all that is within and around me.

Meditation is a surrender. It is not a demand. It is not forging existence your way. It is relaxing into the way. Existence wants you to be. It is a let-go.

Osho

As the years have gone by and my own meditation practice has developed and evolved, I am repeatedly reminded how incredibly powerful the daily practice of meditating really is. Whenever my mood, energy, or inspiration slips these days, it's almost always because my meditation practice has slipped. If you haven't meditated before or think that you can't, it's so much easier than it seems. Most people believe they must silence their mind, but this isn't the case. It's about becoming the observer of your thoughts, rather than consumed by them. When we meditate and a thought comes up, the idea is to simply acknowledge the thought and then allow it to drift away, like it's a cloud in our field of vision. Then we bring our awareness back to the meditation. The more we meditate, the more of a healing, peaceful, and harmonious mind and body we create.

It's important to meditate for as long as feels right for you and as often as feels right, but the main thing is to make sure you are meditating regularly. If you aren't meditating or you don't think it's for you, then perhaps you simply haven't found the right meditation practice for your own needs. There are so many to choose from out there, and not everything works for everyone or they may not be ready for it at that time. If you went to the doctor and they gave you a pill that didn't work, you wouldn't then write off all doctors and medication, would you? Well, the same principle applies to meditating.

Keep trying new ways of meditating until you feel you have found one that works for you. And even after you have found the right one, you may still want to mix your practice up occasionally. I rarely do the same meditation every day; I do whichever ones I feel drawn to. Sometimes these are guided, other times they are silent meditations. I meditate whenever I feel out of alignment, and I know I'm out of alignment when I'm thinking too much, am tired, or things feel like hard work. I also meditate when I'm not sure what to do, feeling out of sorts, or have a question I'd like some insight into. And I meditate also, just because it feels right. What I can promise you, though, is if you fully embody the meditation process and keep yourself grounded throughout, you'll very quickly experience a more harmonious body and mind. Those pesky thoughts and that busy brain will calm down, you'll become more open to new things, and inspiration will come-a-knocking much more often.

Accepting during a meditation practice is incredible. It helps you to get out of your own way, to stop trying to fix, change, and improve, allows the body and mind to teach you whatever it needs to, and move on from whatever is going on for you at that time. It also helps you to realise that all meditations are good meditations.

With some of them you will have lots of thoughts, some not so many, but they are all assisting your wellbeing.

Embrace your inner meditator and assist your inner healer!

I wrote this acceptance meditation for you all (and there is a recording of it available free on my YouTube channel here: https://www.youtube.com/channel/UCocICuTkeW_JaVQpVNbqb_g). If you don't feel any of it fully, then rest there for a little while and be ok with your humanness and/or your resistance around it. Say things to yourself like, it's ok not to fully engage or agree with this. Accept your thoughts around this, but also accept this into your life. Try this or any other acceptance meditation twice a day for 28 days, and see how you feel.

Close your eyes and feel yourself grounded in the seat where you are sitting. Take a few deep, cleansing breaths, up from the earth, through your body, and out your mouth. Place your hand over your heart, and breathe into that space deeply and fully several times. Make sure to expel all your breath each time, and in doing so expelling any doubt, and breathe in total acceptance of where you are right now. With your awareness in your heart, and whilst continuing to breathe in and out of this space, bring these words into your heart:

I am accepting of life's treasures and I know I am one of these.

Life grants me many gifts, which I now see with open eyes and heart,

Life whispers to me and I choose to listen to its messages,

In choosing to accept myself, I accept my life and the magic that will unfold within it.

I accept my past, my history, and what's made me, me.

I accept people's truths, for they represent them – not me.

I speak my truth, for I am worthy of being heard.

I accept that everyone I meet is a teacher for me and my growth.

I accept my body for the magic and miracles it creates every day.

I accept that freedom comes from acceptance.

I rest into a place of acceptance within my heart, and know this is always where everything should end and start.

I accept the honesty and rawness of my life,

I am open to life's lessons, and thankful for my body and mind for looking after me.

I speak my truth; I listen to what's being shared.

I let go of any heaviness I'm carrying, any burdens, mine or of others.

I allow life's love into my life, fully loving what makes me, me.

I let go of life's irritations; I know everything is happening just as it should.

I am connected to life's passions, life's purpose, life's loves.

I surrender to where life is taking me, and I am open and curious of what life will bring.

I give myself permission to live in harmony, to be carried and supported by life.

I am connected to who I am, to my body, to others and life.

In my anchoring. I let go of any residual heaviness holding me back from my power, from realising the totality of what makes me, me!

The greatness of a man's power is the measure of his surrender.

William Booth

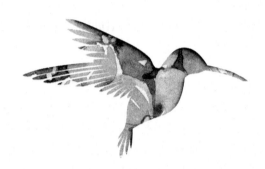

THE BODY'S INVITATIONS TO HEAL

Your body IS NOT against you! Let's get that straight, right from the beginning!

Your body is trying to send you messages to let you know something is out of balance and needs resolving. We can't ignore our way to be well, or even – for the most part – take a pill or potion to make our self well. The symptoms (illness, ailment, or even weight issues) of the imbalance will often go away, but they come back again later on (either in the same format or a similar one). The only way to feel fully well long-term is to see the body's messages (ailments, etc) as invitations to address imbalances.

When we feel our body is against us, we are not only not listening to our body's messages, but we are also causing conflict between the mind and body. Conflict causes dis-ease, which reinforces our ailments or even causes new, additional ones. It does this through many different ways, but one of the main ways is by causing us to go into an underlying anxiety about our body concerns, which triggers or reinforces our fight or flight response (which also reinforces those negative pathways we talked about earlier), and affects the nervous system. This then not only hinders our body's ability to bring itself back into balance, but it starts to have an effect on pretty much all the systems of the body. This is why once we have one ailment, it's more than likely we'll start to get more and more after that. We think this is normal because everyone has ailments, but that's simply because we have all grown up not to listen to our body's messages. When we listen and resolve them, then the body can come back into balance once more.

The same can be said about our negative inner dialogue. Thinking that these thoughts are normal and will just go away or can be ignored, simply does not work. We know this, don't we? The thoughts just snowball. They might get better for a bit here or there, but that's as far is it goes. They always come back, and especially when we aren't in a good headspace. And, then? Well, then they scream at us!

We can be saying dozens of positive affirmations externally each day, but if we are affirming lots of crappy stuff internally then the positive ones we are saying externally aren't really going to get us very far. We need to use the negative inner dialogue to resolve what is asking to be resolved. There is nothing going on in our lives that isn't happening for the purpose of assisting us to grow, wake up, and love a little more.

When we stop looking at our ailments as separate from us, as something to be fixed and using external people or things to 'fix' them, then we can start the process of using these symptoms to resolve the imbalance which they are showing us. They are part of us, they are our mind speaking to us directly, asking us to listen, wanting to be heard. And when we don't listen, our body speaks louder, then louder again until eventually it is shouting at us, and we cannot help but listen. Then we have no choice but to listen, because our ailment hurts us mentally or physically so much by that stage. Wouldn't it be easier if we just learned to listen to its subtle whispering and resolve whatever it is asking of us? It's just a case of learning a new habit, learning to listen, and seeing that our body is not working against us but helping us to come back into balance, to love a little more of ourselves, and to live a little more lightly.

This new pain, illness or condition is not because of your genes, or getting caught in the rain (and 'catching' a cold), or because of your work mate having that tummy bug; it's because of your conditioning!

We believe these things will make us poorly, so they do. We believe it has nothing to do with our inner conflicts, because that's what we have been conditioned to believe. However, ingenious cultures know this is not the case. The ingenious way of thinking is if someone is ill then something must be out of balance within themselves/their lives that is causing the illness. Not who did we pick that bug up from, or did our great aunt have that illness? The science of epigenetics proves that in most cases, genes factor very little in illness, but beliefs, conditioning, and our environment play a major part. Having something run in the family can make us more susceptible to it, but some of this is because we believe it to be the case.

Many ingenious cultures take this a step further when they recognise that an imbalance in our thinking about our present, previous, or future lives, is the real cause of many conditions. Having had first-hand experience of this within my own healing journey and seeing it in the healing journeys of my clients, I can testify to its validity. On one occasion, after 'healing' my digestive system and having done nothing physically to hinder it in any way, it went completely out of control again. I suffered IBS-type symptoms again every day, and was in quite a state. I couldn't understand what was going on or why, but then I listened to the language I was using about my upset digestive system. I was using words like 'it's in turmoil', 'it's really upset', and 'it's irritated'. By following these words/this language I was using, I was able to see that mentally I was in turmoil, really upset, and irritated with a particular thing which was happening in my life at that time. When I resolved the external stress that was causing this imbalance in my body, the digestive issues disappeared pretty much overnight.

There is a mind-based cause behind almost every illness, ailment, or body image issue, which is why some people get the office cold and others don't. Yes, keeping our body fit and healthy helps, but not as much as keeping our minds fit and healthy.

If you have a skin condition, listen to the words you are using about it. Is it making you irritated and/or does it keep people away? Maybe then, someone in your life is irritating you. Or maybe it's a form of protection from something or someone? Weight gain can often be something similar. Does your weight make you feel unattractive, and/or does the food you eat make you feel supported/ protected/feel life's sweetness? If so, then maybe resolving why you feel the need to feel protected, supported, or why you don't feel life's sweetness normally, could be what is causing this imbalance within you.

Listen, really listen, to your body as it speaks to you; listen to your words about your illness and what it is trying to tell you.

Listen, and it will not feel the need to shout at you. Listen, as it creates a better understanding and connection to your body, and with a deeper love for how amazing your body and mind are. Your body speaks words that at the moment you may not hear or understand, but you will, and you will come to realise that the body speaks and it waits for you to listen. When you listen, you will not only resolve the imbalances, but you will deepen your respect and love for all that your body is doing for you each and every day.

And, when we allow ourselves to be conflicted – by not practising acceptance and love in the moment, and not resolving the conflicts/triggers as and when they occur – these conflicts can then become imprinted within us, and cause more current or future health issues to arise. We don't want to do all this work resolving our past issues now, only to not be finding peace with our current issues and having to 'do the work' on these in another five or ten years' time. In the same way that I explained the need to listen to our body and the words it is whispering, the same goes for listening to ourselves and what makes us feel conflicted/ confused/bad in the now.

It can be something as simple as really knowing what our Yes and No to life choices are.

Feel the change within your body now when you think of something bad that's happened to you. Do you feel the tension, the anxiety, and the uncomfortable feeling? Where do you feel it? How does it feel? Is it a colour, or in a certain place in your body? This is your NO; this is your body speaking to you and telling you no, we do not like this.

Now think of something good, do you feel the lightness and the joy in your body? Where do you feel this? How does it feel? This is your body talking to you and telling you YES. When something happens, or you are asked to do something that makes your body react like in the first instance above, then maybe this isn't for you because your body is in a state of conflict. But if the opposite happens, embrace it, enjoy it, and allow it to form part of your journey. It's worth mentioning that sometimes you can feel conflicted through fear of doing something cool. If you do feel fear here, some people would say, 'Feel the fear and do it anyway.' However, I would recommend that you feel into the fear and see where in your life this has stemmed from. Perhaps this situation has manifested to help you resolve a similar situation from your past, or perhaps you are being invited to trust in life more, so you could spend some time resolving this fear and thus stepping through your comfort zone and into your freedom from the fear.

Learn to listen when your body says yes to an event/person/ thing, or no to an event/person/thing. If you really feel you have no choice and need to go with the no, then use the no to help you resolve what your body is asking you to resolve. This way it will not become imprinted on you or cause more imbalances to be resolved moving forward.

For this very reason, do not ignore your inner conflict about anything. Don't push away thoughts or feelings of a negative nature, or that you do not wish to feel. Do not try to mask them with a habit or addiction. Do not think they will simply go away. These feelings are your body speaking to you, telling you that you are out of balance and that something needs addressing. Use these thoughts and feelings to help bring yourself back into balance.

Allow yourself to feel instead of fighting yourself. Feel it, allow it, and then if allowing those thoughts and feelings does not resolve your inner conflict, listen to the language you are using and use it to help you resolve the imbalance within you.

Remember: Your body is not against you! Listen to your body; it speaks a language you may not totally understand at the moment, but the more you listen, allow, and resolve, the healthier, happier, and fulfilled you will be.

If this was happening for me, rather than to me, what would be the blessing?

Lori Cash Richards

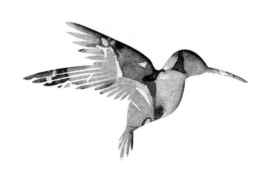

LOVING WHAT'S WITHIN

I believe in the perfection that makes you, you!

I know that you struggle,

I know that you over care,

I know that it hurts

and I know that it often feels like life's not fair.

We are all beautiful beings, pumping blood and producing blood cells (and all manner of other things) every second of every day, travelling on a large magical ball in an infinite and mostly undiscovered Universe trying to find ourselves, when all along we are right here!

Stop fighting, stop resisting, let go, accept, start seeing, start feeling, and take a moment to see how totally and utterly perfect you really are!

Blinded by beauty:

Have you ever noticed when we first see a wonderful landscape, place, or bring a stunning piece of artwork into our home, it is so easy to appreciate its beauty, to see it for what it is? You stop in your tracks, appreciate it in different lights, and see it for the magical gift that it is. But over time, we don't notice these things as much; we almost become blinded by their beauty, as they pass our field of vision so often we no longer even recognise them. Yet their beauty hasn't diminished: it still takes people's breath away every day; it is still appreciated by many, just not so much by us any more. Could it also be possible that this is how we feel about ourselves, that we no longer see ourselves as the magical, beautiful, incredible beings we actually are? We either see ourselves as mediocre or, worse still, as less than others who we perceive to be more magical, beautiful, and incredible than us.

We are no less than we were as a small child. That small child that loved him or herself, their world, and their life. That child was joyous, playful, and totally and utterly accepting of who they were. Why aren't we? Because maybe, just maybe, we are blinded now by our own beauty, by our own beliefs that only allow us to see ourselves through filters; filters we have put in place based mainly on other people's ideas and belief on beauty and love.

When we look on the outside for someone, something, or some event to fill us up, to feel love or to make us happy, this is a wonderful invitation to embody a little more of that exact something within.

We cannot feel the beauty of life's magic when we are always searching for it on the outside, instead of within. When we expect someone to treat us a certain way, to show us love and appreciation, or to make us happy, then it most likely means that we are not feeling this within ourselves. Then, from this place of lack, we become needy, expectant, attached to these people and the outcomes we expect from them. But when we can see that this neediness for someone else to fill this emptiness we feel inside is merely an invitation to fill our own cup, then we can let go of the need for someone else to do this and bring ourselves back into balance. And when we engage with others from this place of fullness, we can have healthier and happier relationships that are not needy, lacking, or depleting for either of us.

What are you looking for in someone else today? How can you invite more of this into your life right now, without being dependent on someone else for it?

Beauty isn't in the eye of the beholder,

beauty is our first breath in the morning,

our skin that not only protects us, but caresses our muscles,

our muscles that propel us to magical locations.

Where we smell, see, hear, and taste life's magic unfolding,

unraveling, and beauty just being,

just resting, and just waiting to be seen.

This same life you are experiencing is within you and flows through

everyone on this extraordinary spinning ball we call home.

The beauty you are blinded to is the beauty of your being,

the beauty of everything, everyone.

The sun does not shine down on you, but out of you.

The woods you walk through grow within you,

the sand you build castles with, forms your bones

and the breath you breathe in your lungs has been breathed

by millenniums of birds, animals, and other human beings all over the world.

The beauty of who you are is without question,

for you are an embodiment of all that is life,

all that is divine and all that is love!

Your greatest gifts are within you, go within!

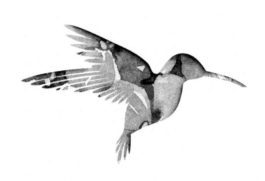

PEACE WITHIN

Belief is one of the most powerful medicines known to mankind!

I wrote the above words, which I knew to be true with illnesses, as I was a living example of this. When I REALLY started to believe I could get well, I started to get well. However, it took me a lot longer to realise that the same words applied to believing that life didn't have to be about fighting myself. I had this underlying belief that because so many people felt the way I did, this must be normal, so I just had to get on with it. NOT TRUE! When I started to believe there must be another way, another way appeared.

Do you fully believe it can be different? Do you *really*? Ask yourself this question and listen to the honest answer. If there's any doubt at all, then this is a wonderful (yes, wonderful) invitation to resolve that belief.

I never thought I'd ever find peace within. Peace within, I thought, was impossible. I'd even convinced myself that the gurus of the world hadn't found it either. That everything was just a big lie to mess with my head. That's one of the reasons I thought there was no point to me or my life, because I thought there was never a way out of this chaos of my mind and life. But my mind was just looking for excuses not to put the work in. I say work so that you know that's how it can feel to start with if you fight it (like I did). But soon you come to realise this is a totally pointless waste of time and that it's just another mind distraction/resistance.

The more I honoured my feelings, myself, and my life, and practised noticing my triggers each day, the easier it became. And now it's just a new unconscious habit I have formed. I could never have imagined that I would go from dishonouring everything I was, to honouring everything I am. But I have, and I love it, myself, and my life, in all its technicoloured glory. For that is now what I see my life as – technicoloured glory in each and every way. No longer is it grey; now it's fluorescent purple, pink, green, orange, yellow, and every other colour there is to see, feel, and embody.

One of my mentors once asked me, what did I desire more than anything? I said peace! He then asked, how much time do you spend on this each day? I was confused; what did he mean? I wanted it every day! He said, how much time do you actually spend on working towards achieving peace each day? I was shocked to realise not very much. Worse than that, I actually spent a good proportion of my day concentrating on all the crap I perceived was upsetting my peace. Sure, I meditated (which had helped tons), but what else was I really doing? And concentrating on the opposite was even worse, because I knew by then that where your attention goes energy flows. So, I was screwing myself over! From that moment, I vowed to take time each day to allow more peace into my world, and to concentrate a little less on what I believed was interfering with my peace.

So, I ask you the same question:

How much time do you spend each day on achieving what it is you want? Not on worrying and stressing about what you don't have, or what you have but don't want. I mean, on what you really want deep down, below the outside influences you think will make you feel a certain way. That feeling deep down; how much time in each day is being spent on it? Really on it? You may find you need to up your game a little, cash in a few chips, spend a bit of time on it, whatever it takes.

Where does the pits of despair really get you? What does the hating yourself really achieve? How is being disgusted with yourself working out for you? How about just for this moment you allow yourself to love rather than hate? How about just for now you let go of judgements, let go of time restraints, let go of all you believe you should be and just be who you are instead? No more fighting, no more conflict, just peace instead. In this moment now, not the past, not the future, in this present moment, right here, right now.

How do we achieve peace within? Firstly, set this as your intention. Fully embody this and know that even in the dark times, this is truly and utterly possible. I know you might not believe me but I've been in the terrible place of feeling my life was pointless, that I was pointless, and that everything about me and my life was disgusting. I also know that when we are not in that dark place, life can be hard; and when in it, life seems completely impossible. It's not. It's just a habit. An old, yet familiar and strangely sometimes comforting place we easily slip back into. But when we are open and loving with ourselves, our lives, and the world, the more this old way of being slips away. The good news is that the more we practise choosing love, the easier the choice for love gets.

So, how do we do this? How do we become more open, and invite more love in? We honour who we are, our thoughts, our feelings, emotions, and choices. We stop fighting life and start honouring it in all its awesomeness. Once we move to this place of love, and away from struggle, conflict, and stress, we achieve not only peace within but peace outside as well. This honouring creates real freedom; freedom from our self-inflicted prison, freedom of choice, and freedom from fear.

How do we practise honouring ourselves and our lives, then?

Notice when you have been triggered. By this I mean, did your boss, friend or family member just say something that hurt or upset you at some level? Don't ignore this, but don't bite back either. Sit with it, don't become consumed by it or by the story of why it is here, just allow it, then honour this feeling/emotion. Honour it because it's part of you and it's your duty to honour you (you can't expect anyone else to do this until *you* do). Honour that feeling, even if it feels like a bad feeling. Now sit with honouring; sit with allowing; and then sit with loving who you are, what's got you here, and that your reaction today was here to teach you a new way of being – not reacting, just being. Doesn't this feel healthier? Doesn't this feel lighter? And doesn't this feel like a much more loving way to be?

The more we practise this new way of being, the less conflicted, stressed out, and anxious we'll be. We'll find we react less to other people and situations. And when we do, we'll know they are just here to help us grow.

Peace won't magically come; it takes practice forming new habits and resolving old patterns. But it will come, and each time it'll get easier. You may find there are times when it's harder again, but know this: these will pass with more ease and grace than they did previously. These hard times are invitations to be more open and accepting, to love a little more, and to resolve whatever triggered you. You'll notice much quicker when you have been triggered the further along this path you have passed. The more time spent being consciously aware of life and its triggers, the easier you'll find your peace in the chaos, and your calm in the storm.

A note on distractions here:

They don't work! Switching on the TV, opening a bottle of wine, eating a takeaway, picking up your phone, or scrolling your Facebook feed, might feel like it's helping at the time, but those feelings won't magically go away of their own accord. They are there for a reason. Listen to them, but don't become consumed by them; allow them and honour them. Distractions only postpone the pain for another time, because in the distraction, nothing has been resolved, no change has been achieved. Whereas, honouring our feelings, thoughts, and self, opens us up, moving from conflict and fear to love and peace. We cannot distract ourselves well, thin, happy or good! Step away from the distractions and feel, really feel, what's going on. Then those feelings will flow, and the distractions can be enjoyed rather than used as a way to sedate ourselves from life.

The secret of happiness, you see, is not found in seeking more, but in developing the capacity to enjoy less.

Socrates

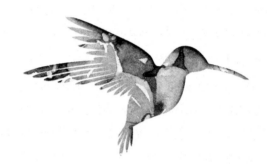

COMPARISON GAME

I am not beautiful like you, I am beautiful like me!

Anonymous

We lose so much of our own power to the comparison game!

We put so much of our own self-worth in the clothes we wear, the furniture we buy, the homes we live in, the latest gadget we own, the cars we drive, the holidays we take, and the jobs and relationships we have. But what if we let this go? What if we stopped judging, comparing, and trying to conform?

1. Write a list of all the things in the last few months that you have purchased (little or large, basically whatever you can remember), which were not a complete necessity.

2. Next to each of these things, write down (and be honest) what feeling, emotion or change in your life you feel this item was supposed to produce. You may need to feel into the time when you were considering buying these things, to get the true answer here.

3. Now write next to each of these if buying this item actually *did* make you feel that way. If it did, is it still doing that now;

if not, how long did that feeling last? A day, a week, or not even that long? Be honest!

4. Now write down everything you are dreaming about purchasing now.

5. Next to each item, write down the feeling, emotion, or change in your life which you expect this to produce.

6. Do you see any similarities?

Are you chasing feeling pretty, confident, worthy enough, full, happy, content with your purchases? Do you see that this is a never-ending cycle of not being and feeling enough?

Don't get me wrong, purchases have their place and it's nice to treat ourselves; in fact, it's an act of self-love sometimes. However, when we are purchasing items from a place of lack and thinking that they will fill us up, then they never will. They cannot; only we can do that.

Learning to love who we are and what we have doesn't mean we never want for anything, or that we go live in a cave somewhere. It simply means we aren't chasing what's on the outside to try and make us happy on the inside.

The same goes for the way we look. When we look at our friends, family, in magazines, on the TV, wherever it is, we very easily slip into playing the comparison game about the way we look, as well as what we have/don't have. That person is thinner than us, has a nice tan, is taller, has a great smile, great hair, lips, etc. When we meet a new person (or even someone we see regularly), we slip easily into judgement about them. Oh look, they are slightly fatter today (yay!), their hair isn't looking as good, they have bags under their eyes, etc. These judgements are a failed attempt to make us feel better about ourselves. And – just as in the previous exercise – if we do feel marginally better, this only lasts a short time and then it's gone again. And, frankly, this is a pretty crappy way to make ourselves feel better about ourselves.

Try not to give yourself a hard time about this, because the judgment game we play has actually served us since the year dot, because it's how we weigh up if something is a threat to us in dangerous situations. It's just now we see perceived threats not just in wild animals and other potentially dangerous situations, but also in all the things out there in the world that trigger our 'not enoughness' or things that may also push us out of our comfort zone.

A much better habit to get into when first meeting someone, is to say the word (in your head is fine) – Namaste. Although there are lots of different takes on this, it basically means 'my soul honours your soul'. By forming this new habit, your brain doesn't so easily slip into the judgment and comparison game when you first meet someone. Instead, there is an instant respect and love for that person and, in turn, for yourself as well.

And remember: Try not to judge your judgement. It's a human response to some old programmes. Honour your humanness and then let it go and it will flow, and you'll have one less thing to make yourself feel bad about. Being human is totally and utterly OK... more than OK!

No-one can hurt you like your own thoughts!

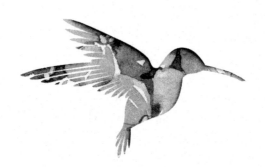

LOST LOVE

I see you in your beauty,

I see the depths of what makes you, you,

I see you standing in your power,

I see you as you reluctantly step up,

I see you for all you have been,

I see deep into those eyes, deep into that soul,

I see you as the world sees you,

as the beautiful, perfect, incredible being you truly are.

I am your heart,

and if you don't see you the way I see you,

then it's just a case of finding your way back home!

I no longer try to be something I am not,

I no longer hide who I really am,

I am who I am and I am perfect,

I am divine, I am love,

Embrace all that makes you, you!

There will only ever be one of you.

One wife/husband,

One mother/father,

One lover,

One teacher,

One student,

One creator,

One lover,

One nurturer and one nourisher within your life, with your past, present and future,

You are divine,

You are love!

Trying to be someone or something you are not, makes for a lot of unhappiness but not much of anything else! When we came to this planet, we loved who we were, totally and unconditionally. We danced, played, sang, and wore what we liked, and it was awesome. We didn't care what we looked and sounded like; we just wanted to play, to have fun, to feel alive. But, unfortunately, we were asked to be quiet, to conform, and to change our very nature of being. We started to lose our individuality and learned that to 'fit in' we needed to be like everyone else. This is so sad! But it can change; we can re-learn what we came here to be, to be heart-centered, happy, and authentic human beings – to be us.

There's a quote I have always loved, even before I really 'got it', and it's from one of my favourite childhood movies (*Highlander*):

There can be only one! How totally, utterly, and completely true this is!

Stop trying to be what you think others want you to be, stop copying, changing, wanting to be anything other than you. For one thing, it's blooming exhausting; for the second, what's the point in trying to be someone else, when the someone else often isn't happy being them, either? If you aren't fully you, you'll attract people that aren't fully them either. People wearing masks, trying to please, not being them, or not being genuine. But when you are fully you, you'll attract others trying to be fully them. You'll encourage healthy, happy, and harmonious relationships and events into your life.

So, how do we learn to love our self again, like we once did as a small child, before we put our self-worth, value, and beauty in the hands of the rest of the world? I have one super-simple, yet beautiful technique for this; one that has had a huge impact on my life and that of the clients I work with. This practice is all about learning to value ourselves, others around us, and life in general. This practice is like a step up from practising gratitude, and is super-powerful.

Self-Value Practice

Firstly, get yourself a small notebook and pen, and leave them by the side of your bed. Each evening before bed (it's best then, as it puts you in a beautiful space for sleep, and allows the subconscious to open up to the work you have done), write down three values. By this I mean, write down what you value about yourself for that day, and/or how you have added value to the world that day.

These things could be as simple as you did the shopping so that someone else in your home didn't have to, or so that you all had food for dinner. It could be you donated to charity, or took something to the charity shop. It could be you sorted out a family member's insurance, or that you didn't shout at someone that you thought deserved it. Or it could be that you told a friend how awesome they were, or how loved someone was. These things of value can be tiny or they can be huge; it really doesn't matter as long as you write them down.

This has a huge impact on your self-worth, but also it makes you realise that a lot of the things which usually stress you out are actually adding value to the world, and how many of them you actually do each day. For instance, you may be stressed out with a family member who keeps messing around your travel plans, but when you list your values you may realise that you have added value to their life because they may not be able to sort these things themselves. For this reason, I highly recommend that you make sure one of your values each day is to do with something which you may be struggling with. It could be that you hate your job, relationship, or home; whatever it is, make one of the values to do with that. And very soon, you will find you no longer feel the same way about that thing, place, or person. You'll see that value has been added to their life, to your working environment, or your community, because of what you have or haven't done that day.

As someone who has spent a lifetime feeling that my life was pointless and not wanting to bother with it more times than I can count, I can tell you this Self-Values Practice is huge! But beware. If you are like me, when you begin it you may find yourself trying to convince yourself that there was nothing of value from your day. I can assure you that's total rubbish (please, don't slam the book shut... stay with me a little longer). You are far too far in your thinking brain and not in your heart, if this is what you are feeling/thinking. I recommend you either do a short, heart-centred meditation at this point, or place your hand on your heart and simply take a few deep breaths in and out of your heart centre. Then, staying in this place, slowly scan your day again and see all the amazing ways you added value to the world today. Especially look at your perceived difficult times throughout the day, and see whose life you added value to then... Because I know you did, and still do!

Replace hate with love, just for today!

Always work with just today, and tomorrow will sort itself out.

This is one of my favourite quotes, I love it so much:

Today you are you! That is truer than true! There is no-one alive who is you-er than you!

Dr. Seuss

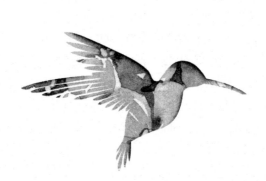

FORGIVENESS

We must be our own before we can be another's.

Ralph Waldo Emerson

The heart retracts when we don't forgive, and then builds walls around itself to 'protect' it from being hurt again. This hinders our ability to hear and receive the love being directed our way, including from our self! Forgiveness is something that is talked about a lot in the spiritual/alternative world, and something I never really got. Why should I forgive what another has done to me, or even what I have done to myself? But not forgiving is like a disease that festers and eats away at us. Often, the person our non-forgiveness is being directed at is not even aware of it, or they are sending more un-forgiveness back at us.

Un-forgiveness is head-based, and forgiveness is heart-based. When you think of that person (or ourselves) that you do not wish to forgive, how does that sit in your body? Does it feel heavy, pressured, stressful, and exhausting? This is what this feeling of un-forgiveness is doing to your body every time you either engage it, or try not to engage with it and push it out of your mind. Instead, why not play with the idea that the way we are reacting to the situation is another invitation from the body to resolve some imbalance within our life? If left unaddressed, this un-forgiveness may imprint on us and cause health issues now and moving forward, due to the conflict it is causing us.

So, use this feeling of un-forgiveness, sit in it, allow it fully within you, allow your humanness; how does that feel? What language are you using? Does this remind you of a time in your past that pushed your buttons the same way? Invite love into the event, invite love into you now, know this is a gift as a lesson to help you grow. You are all you are here to be, right now, right at this moment. Know this!

Forgiving our self and others, allows us to move forward, to become unstuck, to let go of attachments, and to live our life fully. We don't have to start socialising with the people we forgive; we just let go of our attachment to the story/drama around this person or event. Then we won't react in the same way moving forward, and this won't trigger our own doubts, insecurities, and distrust. We are doing the best we can, with what we have, in the time we have it, and we won't all agree or even all get along. But we won't feel triggered by what others are doing, which can have an impact on our own joy!

Ask yourself now: can I forgive this person/myself for this event? Breathe into it, allow it to be, and breathe out the need to be right, to be in control, and to feel heard. Let it go a little more with each out-breath, and breathe in a little more acceptance and love, for yourself and anyone else involved. Where there was once pain and hurt, feel that there is now love and acceptance.

I have a little story of forgiveness I wanted to share with you here, a little story of how forgiving even people who do great wrongs releases us from the self-imposed chains we create when we are stuck in un-forgiveness.

When I was a small child, I was abused by a family friend. This abuse obviously affected many of my choices throughout my life. I refused to be a victim, but I certainly wasn't going to forgive something like this. However, not that long ago, I was working on resolving another whisper from my body when something quite unexpected happened. During this process of resolution, I felt drawn to send love to myself as a child around the age the abuse was going on – which made sense, of course.

When I took myself back to that time, and knelt down in front of myself as a child, and hugged myself and sent unconditional love, my child-self clearly said to me, 'Not me, him.' I instantly knew who my child-self meant and, although there was some hesitation, I knew by then to follow what my heart was telling me. So, although by this time the tears were pouring down my face, I embraced my abuser and sent him all the love I could. As I let go and came back to the present moment, the tears became tears of joy not sadness. I felt instantly lighter, and I knew there had been a big shift within me and a big return of some lost power to me. I fell almost instantly to sleep, and slept all night through. When I awoke, I had a deep love for myself, the world, and even my abuser. I felt no malice, no disgust, distrust or hatred. The love and forgiveness I had shared with my abuser had released me from the inner chains I had created for my own protection. My love of life, trust in life, and energy for life noticeably increased from that day, thanks to releasing my attachment to what had happened to me all those years before.

Forgiveness gives us freedom, and it makes room for more love in our life. Each time we do not forgive, we allow that event/person/situation to imprint on us, to create an imbalance, to affect our health and our freedom to live life fully; we lose a little power (or a lot) with the energy of not forgiving another or – even more – not forgiving our self.

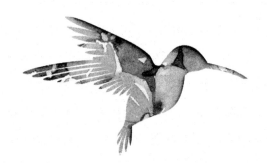

LETTING GO

You will find that it's necessary to let things go, simply for the reason they are heavy.

Anonymous

Why not, just for today, practise letting go?
Let go of that which does not serve you,
Let go of that which weighs you down,
Let go of that which you carry for others,
And let go of expectations now!

Note to self: Stop expecting, start living!

The reason we struggle to let go is because we are attached and/ or resistant to these things, people, and/or events. This isn't a nice place to be in, as we'll often find ourselves being triggered by things which remind us of them. But it is possible to release these attachments and/or resistances, and with each one we release we become more harmonious, more loving, and more understanding or ourselves and others, and more open to the beauty of everything going on around us every day.

So how do we do this?

1. We notice when we have been triggered (someone or something has pressed our buttons). This may take hours or

days, because we are not aware of it when we start down this path. However, with practice, we notice we have been triggered much sooner, and eventually, almost instantly.

2. Then, rather than fighting the energy, emotions, and feelings, we lean into it/them. We feel them, take them on board, and allow them to sit within us. It's our fight with ourselves that causes much of our stress and anxiety, so we are practising allowing instead.

3. Then breathe in and out of the feelings, knowing that they are here to help us, to allow us to let go and move on from the old habit or programme we are playing out because of the trigger.

4. With each in breath in, allow and surrender; and with each out breath, let go of the old habits, patterns, and programmes. Let the tension leave your body, and the love enter your heart.

5. Everything, EVERYTHING is happening just as it should, when it should. And when we learn to let go and embrace and trust in this, we are open to seeing the gifts they bring with them.

We lose much of our power to triggers, habits, and patterns playing out, but we also lose our power to the people and the 'stuff' we hold onto as well. By this, I mean that there may come a time when a person or possession does not serve us any more, and in fact drains our time and energy, but we keep hold of them because of some sort of obligation. We may feel bad for letting them go; they may have been there for us; they have no-one else; or Great Aunt Sally gave it to us.

When you feel your energy drain when you are around someone, or when you pick up an item the same thing happens, then maybe it's time to let them/it go. I know of people who have decluttered their home then found a new partner (because they had energetically made room for that new person in their life). I also know of people who decluttered their office and then lots of new clients came through the doors (for the same reason). I had one client who lost a lot of weight (something they had been trying to do for years) after they cleared away all the clutter in their home.

When we hold onto things which no longer serve us, we don't make room for the things that can. If you want a different kind of energy in your life, then clear away the clutter and make energetic space for it. If you want better relationships, then let go of the ones that take up all your energy. If you want to be more creative, then make space mentally and physically for more creativity. Basically, if you are feeling stuck, there's a good chance the stuckness is because you are holding onto and feeling weighed down by the people and/or possessions around you.

When I recently sold all my possessions and home, I felt lighter in mind, body, and spirit than ever before. I am not suggesting everyone does this (unless they feel called to, ha!), but what I am saying is that a lot of energy/power is lost to holding onto people and things that may not be serving us any more (and probably not serving them either).

Where is your power going? Write a list. Where are your power drainers – a friend, that cupboard under the stairs, your work, or that unfinished book? Can you let go of them, some or all of them? Can you make a conscious plan to slowly clear them away, to give them to another, to let a charity make some money from them, and make energy and room for something else? Really feel into it now. Where are you losing power, and how can you let it go, let it serve another, and make room for more of what can serve you now?

The quote below is a bit extreme, but it resonated so much with me. Our homes – often passed down with possessions gifted to us by loved ones or wills – can form a tomb, where our energy is stuck. Choose carefully what you surround yourself with, and make sure it feels light and not heavy. And, if it's heavy – let it go!

You shall to dwell in tombs made by the dead for the living.

Kahlil Gibran
(when referencing houses)

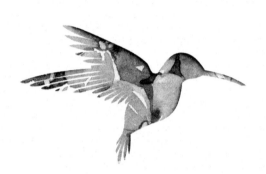

PROTECTION

Thank you, body, for carrying me,

Thank you for being my shelter,

My transport, my protector.

I understand now what you were doing,

I understand now the physical pain was to protect me from the mental pain.

I understand now the perfection of everything you do,

Everything you do, you do for me.

I choose no longer to fight you,

I surrender to your knowing,

I no longer need such protection.

I love you, I love me,

In this love of self, I am protected from all, even myself.

I wrote the above passage when I realised that the headaches I'd been suffering from permanently for 10 years were actually my body protecting me from the pain I had been putting myself through in my mind. When the headache was as intense as it could get, I couldn't think any more due to such intense pain. So, it worked!

Early in our healing journey, we often figure out that our mind and body have been trying to protect us against trauma, abuse, events, places, and people. We can often put on weight or start suffering from a skin condition to protect ourselves against abuse or bullying, for instance.

What sometimes takes a little longer to realise is that, most of the time, that protection is from our self. From our own thoughts and feelings. We are often bought up to feel we are less than others if we haven't achieved what they have, aren't as popular as others if we aren't as slim or pretty, and worthless if we don't fit in with the crowd. This means that at a young age we are already giving ourselves a hard time, trying to conform, and trying to *not* be us. The mind and body then try to protect us from our own thoughts, just like they would if there was an outside attack from someone else. This might appear in the form of weight gain (or loss), skin conditions, tummy upsets or constipation, memory issues, headaches, or a whole host of other ailments.

The greatest threat to us, is us! There is nothing outside of us that can threaten our health and wellbeing as badly as our own thoughts. They are super-strong, ninja thoughts, so choose them wisely.

Have you noticed that some people seem to be able to stay healthy even though endless, crappy things are happening to them? It's because these people don't think about these things in the same way that the rest of us do. They see them, feel them, and then move on from them. Becoming stuck in the crappiness does not serve any of us. When we accept where we are, we can move through it and use it as fuel to empower us along our journey. But when we start to think the world is against us and that all these bad things always happen to us, we start to shut down, slip into the fight or flight response again, and become stuck in a very negative way of being. When we are in that position, we don't see life's possibilities, life's invitations, and life's beauty, and we start to need protecting from our own hurt, pain, and thoughts.

Everything that is happening to us right here, right now, is to help us grow. I know it doesn't feel like it at the time, but if you keep that in mind eventually you'll see through the pain and find the gifts instead.

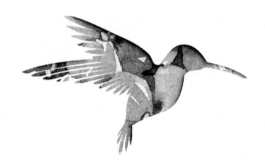

LOVING KINDNESS

When I loved myself enough I began leaving whatever wasn't healthy. This meant people, jobs, my own beliefs and habits – anything that kept me small. My judgement called it disloyal. Now I see it was self-loving.

Kim McMillen

If we heard someone talk to another the way we talk to ourselves, we'd be shocked, appalled, and maybe even disgusted. So, why do we allow ourselves to speak to ourselves, about ourselves, in this way? Because we haven't been taught to love and respect ourselves; we've been taught that we are not enough, we need to conform, and we need to do better!

However, when we speak to ourselves in a more loving way, when we make a conscious effort to be kinder to ourselves, things change. If we speak to ourselves in the way we would want to be spoken to by someone else, then that whole relationship changes. If we speak in a more loving way to the body parts we dislike, our whole relationship with our body changes. Thank your belly for carrying and protecting your beautiful children, or for all the amazing meals it has allowed you to enjoy, or all the laughs it has been part of in the pub over a beer.

Find something good – a memory or an event that each body part has been involved in creating. Find ways to talk to and create a healthy relationship with the body parts you dislike the most. And, consider this: our skin replaces itself once a month; our stomach lining every five days; our liver every six weeks; and our skeleton every three months. Now, that's amazing! Cultivate kindness, for it cultivates love and allows us to live more fully in the knowing of our wholeness!

Cultivate a dialect of kindness between you and your body, and know that you are not only creating a more loving space to live in, but that the energy which was once wasted on hating who you are, will go into loving you and your life instead.

Here's a great (and really simple) loving kindness kind of question which I think is really important to make consciously kind choices for ourselves and not the distracted, sleepwalking kind of choices that keep us where we don't desire to be.

In my last book, *Cleanse,* I asked readers to ask themselves: 'Is this nourishing or nurturing for mind, body or spirit'?' But I've shortened it for you here. Whenever you have a choice to make, ask: 'Will this make me feel good about myself?'

It basically asks you whether whatever you may be about to do is going to make you feel good or bad about yourself. This is a great question to ask ourselves, because it makes us conscious about our choices. And it means we may not take the easy train to distraction with the next sugar, booze, or person fix, as these fixes fade quickly and often make us feel worse afterwards. Instead, this question provides us with a few moments of consciousness to consider what our next choice might bring us, allowing us to practise loving kindness for ourselves. This then goes on to form new healthy and kind habits.

The longest and most important relationship you will ever have, is with yourself. Make it the relationship that counts, make it the one that empowers, that inspires, that creates, that births, that nourishes and nurtures, like no other. If we make it the only one we really need, then when we meet someone else who complements our own relationship with our self, we will find that we do not 'need' this person, we will not 'depend' on this person, and we will not be 'attached' to this person.

Practising loving kindness towards compliments/gifts is also just as important. Often, when someone pays us a compliment, we brush it off, turn away from it, or put it down. Firstly, that is not a kind way to accept a gift such as this from another well-meaning and beautiful soul. Secondly, you are not being kind to yourself. Compliments really are gifts in the way of words, and should be accepted as such. Energetically, every time we block a compliment, we block the love, kindness, and compassion behind it. Eventually, that person will stop giving us these gifts.

So, when we receive these beautiful gifts from another, remember that they wouldn't say these words if they didn't believe them, and it's a great honour that they are sharing some of their love and energy with us – and let's try not to block that. Once you realise this, you will easily feel the change in energy as you go from putting up barriers and deflecting these gifts, to openly letting them in along with the people who shared them.

The more love and beauty we accept, the more we will attract, as we raise our vibration rather than blocking this beautiful energy from us.

Because she competes with no-one, no-one can compete with her.

Lao Tzu

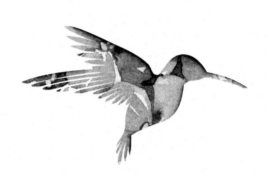

CONNECTEDNESS

When did we start losing touch with ourselves, each other, and this world? When did it become acceptable to be consciously unaware of everything? How did this happen?

Actually, who cares? The fact of the matter is, we are disconnected from our bodies, each other, and the planet. We are not aware of what we put into our bodies, where it comes from, how it's produced, or where. We live in a bubble, assuming this bubble protects us from harm. But the bubble is one of the most harmful things we carry with us. Without the connection to our own bodies, each other, and life, we start to feel lonely, stuck, isolated, disconnected, disjointed, and lacking.

How can we live a healthy and energised life if we are unwilling to connect with, listen to, and learn from our bodies? How can we have nourishing relationships, if we are unwilling to connect fully with love instead of fear? How can we expect things on this planet to change, if we will not connect with all life that lives on it? We cannot. Connection is part of what makes us *us*. It's believed in many indigenous cultures that the lack of connection to ourselves, each other, and the planet, is behind many modern illnesses.

Even if you can't bear (yet) to do any of the lovey-dovey stuff in this book, you could spend some time connecting back to self; take some time each day to focus on re-establishing a connection with your body, centering, grounding, and going within. If we are not fully present and centered within ourselves, then the other beautiful stuff we are doing for ourselves will not work effectively. It's the number one thing to focus on from this book!

Consider consciously creating a healthier dialogue with yourself, meditate regularly, say hi to your neighbours, walk barefoot, think about where your food is coming from, and whether you can be part of the process of nurturing better practices by the shopping choices you make. See how important your function within this world is. How beautiful life is when you consciously connect with it.

Breathe in and breathe out from your heart, then allow this energy of the heart and your breath to connect you with the things, and people, and places around you. Slowly expand this feeling out to your local environment, then town, city, country, continent, and then the whole planet, and the whole Universe. Be at one, connected to all that is; you are part of this magic, you are part of this beauty, you are both a divine being and the Universe as a whole. As such, you can never be alone; you have simply lost your connection to what is true. Bring this connection to everything slowly back into your heart, and rest in the deep feeling of connection.

Take some time now to rest your awareness in your body, and then slowly move your fingers over your hands, then arms, then shoulders and neck, face, head, chest, breasts, stomach, genitals, legs, feet and toes. Where did you find this difficult? Why do you think this was? Have you been trying not to connect with that particular area (ignoring or disliking it)? Now try again, but with the curiosity of a small child as they play, learn, and appreciate. Gently move your fingers over your body again, as if feeling it like a child would, with wonder, joy and curiosity. Play with the rolls of fat, smile at them, appreciate the smoothness of your skin, the life your body has experienced, and the tapestry that makes it what it is. How does that feel now? Keep playing, especially with the areas you struggled with before. Look at them now, not as an adult with a lifetime of dishonoring and disrespecting behind you, but with a child's wonder of the world. You are beautiful and your body is amazing; it wants to be heard, connected with, and honoured. Keep playing, exploring, and connecting back with your body, and build a healthier relationship with it and with your life.

Dance is one of the oldest and most effective ways to connect with ourselves, our community, and even Mother Nature. It is nourishing, nurturing, expressive, healing and, of course, a great form of exercise. We don't have to join any special groups or even know how to dance, all we need to do is move to the music that's playing inside or outside of our own heads (by this, I mean there doesn't even have to be music to dance!). Just move, sway, go crazy, whatever feels good, and don't worry about what you look like, just what you feel like. Feel the music of life as it beats inside. Become completely consumed by it, allow your mind to take a back seat and your spirit to come forward, to play, to be curious, to move through you, and to connect you deeply to your soul.

If you feel silly doing this, or are not sure where to begin, then start by shaking your body. This helps you to release any tension within the body, to let go of your apprehensions, and starts to get the energy flowing.

This is a good place to start if dancing makes you feel a little too vulnerable:

1. Stand up, take your shoes and socks off, and centre yourself. Then (if you can) go outside and make contact with the earth, supported by Mother Nature.

2. Shake your right foot; shake, shake, shake that foot out as much as you can.

3. Shake the left foot; shake, shake, shake that foot as much as you can.

4. Now shake your right leg, all the way up, shake it out, really get moving.

5. Do the same with the left leg, shake it.

6. Now shake your booty, wiggle it, really shake it, just like a very, very happy dog!

7. It's time to shake your pleasure centre now, shake it like there is no tomorrow. Feel all your tensions and apprehensions being shaken away.

8. Shake that belly and back now; really shake that beautiful belly; shake, shake, shake it.

9. Shake that chest, stick it out, shake it around, feel the chest expanding and opening. Give it a good old shake.

10. Shake those shoulders out now, really shake them, let go of all the tension you are carrying there; shake, shake, shake.

11. Shake your right arm, all the way down, shaking the hand

and fingers at the same time; shake it all, let it go loose, shake it.

12. Now do the same for the left arm, hand and fingers, give them a good old shake.

13. Shake your neck and head, shake them free from thinking. Shake, shake, and shake.

14. Now shake the whole body out, go mad, just shake it all, jump around if you want, lay down and shake your limbs, shake until you can't shake any more.

15. Feel that energy being released, feel the connection between every part of your body, and know that all areas of your body have equally been part of this. Shake it!

16. This whole process can take as little as 5 minutes or as long as you like; just do what feels right.

Now, if it feels okay, move on to dancing.

1. Put some slow music on to start, and slowly move/sway.

2. It's not really dancing to start with, it's more like waving and weaving, allowing your body to flow with the music.

3. Let go of how you look; this is all about how you feel.

4. Allow all areas of your body to wave and weave with the music, to flow and to connect, both to you, to the music, and to the world.

If you want to step it up a gear, you can now speed up the music.

1. Move your body to the music, to the beat, don't choreograph it, let go of how you look, just move that body, all of it.

2. Move all your limbs, your neck, and your head. Feel the beat of the music and life as you connect with it. Become totally absorbed by it, by life, and by the love within each and every thing on this planet.

3. Dance, move, wave, and weave for as long as feels good.

4. When you are done, power down again. Come down to slower music and slower movements, and then to gently shaking out your body again. Start with the feet and work your way through the shake-down (as above), from start to finish.

5. Now lay on the floor and feel the rhythm and connection to life within you. Simmer in the afterglow of your dance with yourself and life. Allow yourself to be grounded with Mother Nature, and just be!

Connecting back to Mother Nature – Earthing/ Grounding

We were born on the earth, ate, slept, and lived almost all of our lives connected to the earth. It's only in recent years that this is no longer the case, and this disconnection from the earth, from Mother Nature, is now manifesting itself in various illnesses – both mental and physical.

Our disconnection with Mother Nature is like being disconnected to part of ourselves. Not only that, but our increasing connection to technology causes electromagnetic stress and this can manifest as anything from headaches and memory issues to muscle problems and fatigue (see my first book *Living a Life Less Toxic* for more about this). Luckily, though, re-connecting is simple. Get out in nature, walk barefoot, paddle in the sea, hug a tree (yes, tree hugging works), get as much skin as possible in contact with as much nature as possible. This will earth/ground you, which will not only help to reduce the effects of our technological age but it will also connect you back to life. This has a huge impact on our mental and physical health.

> *I believe there is a subtle magnetism in nature, which, if we consciously yield to it, will direct us aright.*
>
> **Henry David Thoreau**

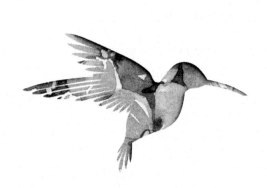

THE SANCTUARY WITHIN

My friend, Jane A. Cormack, in her book *Language of the Feminine,* invites you to create a space within that you would want to come home to. A happy, clean, safe place that is filled with its own unique expression and energy. She says, imagine nourishing your inner environment so your 'home' works efficiently. This is what I mentioned in the chapter Consciously Creating Change, earlier in this book. Thinking about how we are fueling our inner sanctuary allows us to consciously create changes that fuel it better. Distracting, ignoring, and busying does not! If we don't fuel it well, we often find we do not want to be in the body we are in, and it may not be performing and looking how we would like it to.

When I mention fuel, I don't mean just food, although this plays an important part. What plays a bigger part is what we are doing at a mental and spiritual level. Thus, things like meditations, exercise, tapping/EFT, down-time, walking, writing, journaling, talking, learning, growing, loving, and even the relationships we have, are all fuel in some way.

I want you to ask yourself this right now: How are you fueling yourself right now? What or who are you drawing on for power?

131

Are you drawing on power from certain people around you? Are you fueling yourself badly? Or are you not really fueling yourself at all? Is your power fueling other people?

Be honest, be open, and be true to you. This will help you to see where changes could be made. Choose a healthier way to fuel your body and your life, and build a kinder and stronger sanctuary within.

As I mentioned earlier, our thoughts form part of the fuel for our bodies, minds, and lives. So, with healthier and more loving thoughts, we'll have healthier and more loving bodies and lives.

In doubt? Feeling fat? Confused? Not feeling enough? Whatever that pesky thought is, do something for me, for you, for your life. Rather than becoming consumed by that thought again and again and again, bring your awareness to the space you occupy, not to the body part you dislike or the conflict within your life. Just simply to the space you occupy. You won't fix the 'issue' by thinking about it; if that worked, then everything in your life would be peachy now, wouldn't it? Come out of the thinking and into just 'being'; stop putting your attention on what you *don't* want and allow this peace of awareness in.

When we are in this space, we are no longer in conflict, no longer creating dis-ease, and no longer fighting that long, tiring, and endless battle with ourselves. When we become consciously aware of our thoughts and actions, they don't run the show any more. Instead, we can see the crazy brain in action and choose to simply not engage with the craziness any longer. When we stop trying to 'fix' ourselves and start instead to accept, honour, and nourish ourselves, then we create a beautiful inner sanctuary and we can create whatever we want from there.

So, before trying to figure out our purpose, our health, our love life, career, or anything else, let's build our inner sanctuary and from there everything else will flow much more easily. We have become obsessed with changing ourselves – even if that's just for our health – but our commitment instead should be to become centered, grounded, and loved from the inside out, then the rest will sort itself out.

I feel lost within a body that doesn't work right.

Lost within a world that doesn't see me.

Lost within a life that's doesn't matter.

Lost within relationships that don't understand me.

I am stuck, I am fearful, and life is a mystery.

I look on the outside for what I know is within.

I need to fix this feeling.

I need to be OK somehow.

What's fueling me now?

What's giving me power?

How's my environment within?

When life is just crazy, can I safely retreat inside?

Can I build a sanctuary I'd want to live in?

Can I build this sanctuary, right here within?

The greatest gift you have is your life!

Over the last few years, my eyesight has become progressively worse. Most people think this is normal as we get older, but for me it was a sign that something was out of balance within me. It was an invitation to dive into that perceived health ailment and see what I could do. So, from a place of open-hearted awareness, I asked myself what this was here to show me. I clearly heard: 'whilst you are unwilling to see yourself, so are your eyes.'

Being unwilling to see ourselves, disconnects us from part of who we are. It dishonors and disrespects who we are, and creates a body and mind in disharmony, one that easily sits in dis-ease thus creating disease. To create a place of harmony, we must create a place of honor, respect, and love.

If you don't feel ready right this moment to see and honor all of you, then set an intention and give yourself permission to be open to doing this moving forward. This sends a powerful message to the subconscious that you are ready for change. Be open to being open. Use this as a mantra, an affirmation, a Tapping/Emotional Freedom Technique (EFT) routine, or even during meditation, but either way be open to being open, to start to unravel your previous habit of pretending parts of you are not there, or that they are unimportant. All parts of you and your life are equally important, deserve equal respect, and to be held kindly within your inner sanctuary.

Lastly, does your outer sanctuary reflect your inner sanctuary, or how you would like your inner sanctuary to be? This means, is it calm, relaxed, nurturing, and nourishing? Or is it cluttered, busy, and overwhelming? Creating an outer sanctuary that is somewhere we feel able to slow down, relax, and find peace, will help us to do just that. Consider what items you have around you that don't encourage this, which items keep you attached to past events, and which items could better serve someone else. Start making more room on the outside and you will create more room on the inside. When we let go and clear away physically, we are more able to do the same mentally.

> *Three rules of work: out of clutter find simplicity; from discord find harmony; in the middle of difficulty lies opportunity.*
>
> **Albert Einstein**

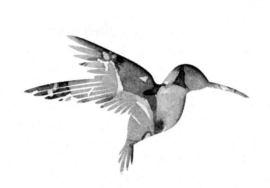

LOVING THE SKIN YOU'RE IN

The curious paradox is that when I accept myself just as I am, then I can change.

Carl Rogers

If I said you had a beautiful body, would you hold it against me?

**David Bellamy
(The Bellamy Brothers)**

The fact of the matter is, many of us probably would. But why? Why have we have become so disconnected from the beauty of who we truly are? From the magic of our skin, our hips, the smell from our nose, the hearing from our ears, the sight from our eyes, the skeleton and muscles that hold everything in place. How is it that we've become obsessed with what these things look like, rather than what an amazing job they do for us each second of each day?

For most of my life, I have neither loved nor respected myself nor my body. I have used and abused it myself, and allowed others to do the same. I then spent years disgusted with my body. Every time I looked at my body or tried to connect back with it in any way, I would feel shame, disrespect, and disinterest (plus, I always then assumed others felt the same way about me).

It's no surprise then that by hating my body in this way and by allowing myself to disconnect from it, I collected many health ailments (including finally being housebound with ME/CFS). But what I didn't quite grasp was that these health ailments were based on my hate of my body and not on what food I was eating, exercise I was doing, or what products I was using. Don't get me wrong. I made huge leaps and bounds in recovering full health by addressing these things, but what really returned me to full health – both mentally and physically – was resolving the conflict I felt about me!

It's easy to become blinded by the beauty of who you are. We live such busy lives, and much of the time we feel the need to 'be more', 'achieve quicker', and 'look better'. At one time, we all did believe ourselves to be beautiful. When we were small children, we were fascinated by who we were, our own reflection, and the beauty of life. But, as we moved through life, we slowly lost this amazement with everything, including ourselves. Not only that, but many of us were taught that it's wrong to love ourselves or selfish to spend too much time thinking about ourselves and our lives.

I wanted to share with you a poem I wrote to my body...

> *I spent a lot of life hating you*
>
> *and I thought you hated me back,*
>
> *you wouldn't do what I wanted*
>
> *I mean, for instance, you were fat.*
>
> *But now I've come to see,*
>
> *you were simply inviting me,*
>
> *to wake up to the truth of who I really am.*

But I listened not,

I heard nothing,

I saw only what I wanted to

and ignored all but that.

Your callings fell on deaf ears,

I looked for happiness on the outside, rather than within.

Slowly I realised this wasn't the way,

for it hurt, I hated, and it kept me trapped.

I felt I was in a never-ending battle,

a battle I could not possibly win,

for I was leading the fight on both sides of the battlefield within.

I reminded myself I did not come here to hate myself,

I did not come here to fear, to hurt,

and to let my life slip away like that.

I reminded myself I am love, and love is always enough.

A gift of light, a gift of growth, and a gift of life.

I chose to surrender; each and every day, I do the same.

I surrender the fight and I surrender to the love and to the light.

The magic of my life is the greatest gift I've been given,

I pledge to honour this, respect this, and know

when I am not, I have simply lost sight of what and who I am, for
what I am not!

How do you love a body you hate? How do you accept what feels far from great? How can you be all you can be? Who the hell are we? These are all the questions I asked myself; they may be like the questions you are asking yourself.

In answer to these questions, I wrote, I journaled, and I meditated, and then I surrendered to what this was all here to teach me. What I got back (in abundance) was:

Calm Loving Respect!

I invite you to do the same. I invite you to be totally open to the writings and ideas in this book and others, and to spend time every day surrendering to what this is all here to teach you. Maybe what you get back is different from what I wrote above, but many of us are missing these three simple things!

Calm:

We need calm if we want to be in a healthy, harmonious, and happy state. To be open to what our body is inviting us to resolve. To make the time to meditate, surrender, and be open to the lessons we are here to learn. Invite calm into each of your days; make time and space to create a little harmony. Calm seems like such a simple concept, but it's also so profound. If you do nothing else for yourself but allow calm into your daily routine, you will very quickly reap the benefits and sow new seeds for a more harmonious you.

Loving:

Obviously loving will create more love, but it's the loving of yourself that does this, not the loving of others or their loving of you. This can fade, change, be borrowed or evolve, but the love you hold for yourself will allow you to live in harmony with many perceived hurts and heartaches. I invite you to step off the hate train for a second, and to fully immerse yourself in the beauty of that amazing body you are in. Every second of every day it's pumping blood around your body, it's making your limbs move, allowing your lungs to breathe, and giving you the beauty of touch. Really think about that for a second; isn't it totally incredible? Even if you dislike your body in some way or it's not as healthy as you would like, you have to admit it's still doing an amazing job every second of every day, isn't it?

Respect:

It's easy to disrespect our bodies. They don't look the way we want them to, or are not performing at the rate we wish them to. These sorts of thoughts and feelings haven't got us anywhere, though, have they? How about just for today you play with the idea of respecting this incredible vessel in which you are travelling through this amazing Universe? Your body has been protecting you, not just from the outside world but from the inside projections, fears, and worries you have been focusing on for much of your life. It's been doing an amazing job, considering what you have been throwing at it, wouldn't you agree?

You may disrespect your body, but what if I told you it's ok to let go of those old thoughts and feelings now, that it's ok to move on? These times taught you what you needed to learn, they were part of creating the path to where you are now. But it's time to move on! Just sit with this for a second. How does replacing disrespect with respect feel? No-one said you had to hold on to these feelings, these wrongs, this disrespect. You can literally choose healing over heartache now! Ask yourself now: 'Can I let go of disrespecting myself'? Feel the answer, embrace it, and take some deep breaths. You may have to ask yourself this time and time again, but each time it will be a little easier and each time you'll notice sooner that you have slipped into respect. And, if you cannot let go of this now, then ask yourself this: 'Can I be open to letting go of disrespecting myself, moving forward?' And send that powerful message to the subconscious mind that things are on the move, things are going to be changing, and you are becoming ready to let go.

Don't be a weight watcher:

For those wanting to lose weight, it's amazing how when you fully embody calm, loving respect, the weight simply balances out at a happy, healthy place. This is because we are no longer in a fight or flight/adrenal response, so we are not suffering from underlying stress and anxiety. Instead, we are creating a place of nourishment and nurturing for our body and mind. We are no longer reinforcing the very things we do not want with our thinking, but we are loving what we do have instead. We are also allowing ourselves to let go, lightening the load mentally, which then has a huge impact physically. I have lost count of the number of clients whose weight has dropped off when they started to resolve and let go of how they felt about themselves and their lives. What we focus on flourishes! For that reason, don't be a weight watcher, as this only creates more weight for most of us. Focus on the opposite and create the opposite. Focus on calm, loving respect, and that's what will be created within body and mind, instead of heaviness, heartaches, and dislike.

Apart from some incredibly unhealthy times in my life when I was suffering from a health condition or I was partying way too hard, I have always hated my body – and in particular, my weight. It wouldn't matter that other people said that they thought I was slim; I didn't, and I would do my best to cover it/me up. It wasn't until I started REALLY loving, respecting, and nurturing myself and my body, that my body in turn did the same back. Not just through changes in my health, but also in the shape and size of my body. The more I loved my body for its magic, its beauty, and its curves, the more my body became beautiful to me. What you focus on really does flourish!

Wholeness is not achieved by cutting off a portion of one's being, but by integration of the contraries.

Carl Jung

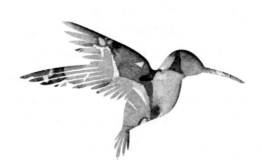

NOURISHING TIMES

Here's some of my top tips for eating better. It's not the next fad diet, programme, or detox. It's honest, easy, and feels amazing:

> ➢ Eat high vibration foods (as close to their natural state as possible and grown and produced in a natural and sustainable way)

> ➢ Eat the rainbow (the more colourful the better)

> ➢ Eat real (if it doesn't look similar to how it came out of the ground, tree, animal, then it's likely been messed about with)

> ➢ Eat, cook, and shop consciously

Listen, really, really listen to your body! What's it telling you about your food and drink choices? Just because everyone else feels regularly bloated, tired, constipated, got the runs, has a headache, and lives on their next caffeine hit, that doesn't make it ok. It may have become the norm, but that doesn't mean it should be your norm.

Make conscious food choices. If you are craving a sugar or caffeine fix, why is this? Feel into it. Could it be that the craving is because you are searching for the sweeter things in life? Are you needing some comfort? Some support or protection? If you can feel into the feelings behind the cravings, you can use the cravings as a way to resolve emotional imbalances.

Binge eating is an invitation to do just this. With food, simply ignoring away the cravings (because you are on yet another diet or programme) does not work. You already know this, right? Willpower only works short term. You may lose a little weight for a short while but, according to research, 97% of people put that weight back on again – and, more often than not, put on even more weight. Why is this? It's not because they are lazy or lack willpower! It's because the underlying emotions behind the food cravings haven't been addressed. Our bodies are always giving us messages to address imbalances within our thinking. Most ailments are, in fact, symptoms of an imbalance in our thinking. Once we can see them in this light, we can 1) stop falling into the stress response about these ailments (which makes them and other issues worse; and 2) move through them much quicker, because we see the learnings and opportunities, and the ways to resolve them with ease. Our vibration and energy around our eating and body image also becomes much better. And, as we know, like attracts like.

For instance, at the time of writing this book, I have started craving walnuts and cauliflower a lot. So, I am going with this, because my body obviously needs whatever is in these foods at this moment. Also, they say that foods which look like different parts of the body are good for that part of the body. As both of these foods look a little like brains, I figure I am in need of assistance in that department whilst writing this book. So, this book comes to you on walnut and cauliflower power!

If I wasn't listening to my body's needs (like I used to), then I would ignore these strange cravings and would be eating masses of other rubbish instead, whilst my body tried desperately to be sated by what I was feeding it. This is often the case when we do not eat a diet high in nutrients. We can often find we are bingeing on rubbish in our body's attempt to find the nutrients it requires to function. But if you eat a diet high in nutrients, this is less likely to happen and, in fact, you will likely eat much less, because your body is getting what it needs from what you do eat. This is why I recommend to 'eat the rainbow', because in that way we increase our chances of getting everything we need from our food through eating a good variety of colourful foods, which are generally high in many different nutrients.

Comfort Eating:

We've all done it! We might not have called it comfort eating, we may have fought it or fallen foul of it, but it's had us all in its grip at some point. But why? Well, there are several reasons actually, and they will differ not only from person to person, but from week to week. Basically, what it all boils down to is trying to change how we are feeling through our food. It's a distraction mechanism, or a way of filling ourselves up when we aren't feeling very full in our lives.

Sometimes there are deep habits around our food choices, based on the need for support, comfort, or protection, from when we were a child (and/or older). This can mean that if we were abused, we may (at a subconscious level) overeat to form a protective layer around us and/or to try to make ourselves feel unattractive to others. Or if we didn't get the comfort we craved for as a kid, we may search out comfort in something we always do get it from – food! Or if we have never felt supported by our family and/or friends, we may look for that support in food because it doesn't make us feel alone.

There is also comfort eating when we are trying not to feel whatever emotions we are currently experiencing. We humans have become masters of distraction, and trying not to feel. But it never works for very long; these emotions are here to be felt, to be honored, and to be resolved. **When we don't allow ourselves to feel all our feelings, then we will fill up on food instead**. Why? Because of the chemical reactions in the body, food can easily change how we feel (both emotionally and physically).

I have noticed a long-standing habit of mine is that I don't comfort eat when I am upset (I tend to starve myself in these times instead), but I can easily comfort eat when I am not being true to myself. When I cannot fully be me (for whatever reason I have thought up this time, ha!) I will reach for food. That's because I am trying not to feel those feelings, trying not to be all of me. I hadn't actually realised I was doing this until I felt into why I was eating so much again one time. Even though it was good foods, it was masses and masses of good foods. When I felt into this (and really listened to my inner voice/messages), I realised that I was trying to dull myself down for someone else. Yep, these things still come up, even when you have done lots of 'work' on yourself. It's not a bad thing; it's just my mind and body talking to me, sending me messages that there is an imbalance in my thinking. Remember: Everything really is happening for us, not against us!

When we are trying to change how we are feeling, we will often use the things that we think have worked for us before. This might be food, drink, drugs, sex, exercise, people, or something else. But we cannot distract ourselves healthy or different, so the cycle will continue. It may get better for a short time with the most recent distraction(s), but that's all that happens. It disappears for a short while and then comes back again, and usually with a big kick up the butt.

The next time you become aware that you are comfort eating, feel into the feelings you are having (not the oh-my-God-this-cake-rocks feelings), the feelings underneath what you are doing. By feeling into it, I mean:

- ➤ Rest into how you are actually feeling; take some quiet time.
- ➤ Put your hand on your heart.
- ➤ Rest your awareness there, and breathe in and out of that space.
- ➤ Now whilst in the heart space, and without going off searching for answers, ask yourself the following questions:
- ➤ How am I actually feeling?
- ➤ What is underneath that feeling?
- ➤ And underneath that?
- ➤ And underneath that? And so on.
- ➤ Keep going until it's all out. Jot it all down, if you need to.
- ➤ Then allow the basic raw feelings in. Embrace them and your humanness.
- ➤ Be ok with having this human experience, and grateful for the opportunity to embrace a little more of yourself.

➢ Now be ok with having the feeling(s); you are human, these are ok, you are more than ok for having them.

➢ Breathe in and out of these feelings, caressing and embodying them, allow them to be within you.

➢ Don't get caught up in the story of why you feel the feelings are there. Just allow them to reside there. Honour and respect them.

➢ When you feel ready, take a few deep breaths to centre and ground yourself, and now see if you want that distraction. Or if you still do, are you in a better place to enjoy it, rather than using it as a distraction/way to change how you are feeling?

When we are no longer conflicted by the feelings we are having, we can let go of the need to try to change them through food, and simply enjoy the process of eating and fuelling our body in the right way.

Another interesting thing that happened to me when I was overeating, was that my head (and nutrition training) told me I was probably deficient in something or another, and this was my body's way of searching for it. When this continued, I realised that I had been trying to resolve the overeating from my head and not from my heart. But when I listened to my heart, I got a true and nurturing response and was able to feel the emotions I had been trying not to feel. This then reduced my need to fill up on food I did not need. It's another great example of how listening to the heart, rather than the head, helps create a harmonious life.

If you want to eat better, try adding good foods in before you start removing the 'naughty' ones. When you start adding more nutrient-dense foods, you will feel full up quicker, as your body is getting the nourishment it requires. So, maybe add a healthy juice to your daily routine, or chia seeds into your porridge oats, or nuts and seeds into your salads, or seaweed into your meals.

My favourite, and probably one of the best things you can add to your diet, are fermented foods and drinks. By fermented, I do not mean pickled. I mean traditionally fermented foods, like unpasteurized sauerkraut, kimchi, kefir, and kombucha. These foods and drinks are highly nutrient and probiotic dense, so they detox the body, improve energy, hormones, mood, memory, and the immune system, and help you to absorb nutrients from other foods and drinks which you consume. They are great to have on the side of your take-away or other 'naughty' foods, to help you process them easier, get more nutrients from them, and to detox afterwards. WINNER!

You can find lots of recipes for these on my website and in my two previous books. Not only will you be loving yourself from the inside out by eating them, but they will improve how you feel about yourself and your life, because they assist in healing the digestive system – where a good proportion of our serotine and other happy hormones are produced. I saw fermented foods referred to as Nature's Prozac in a magazine I recently read. Go, fermented foods!

Don't give yourself a hard time for dipping into the biscuit tin (or whatever is your go-to comfort food). When we give ourselves a hard time for eating the 'naughty' foods, or not exercising or making other healthy choices for ourselves, what we actually do is reinforce the very thing we do not want to do or be. When we give ourselves a hard time for behaviour like this, we cause underlying stress and anxiety within ourselves. That then creates more unhappy emotions and hormones, which leads us to trying to switch these off or change these feelings in some way, usually through food and drink again.

For instance, we convince ourselves that because we have fallen off the wagon (so to speak), we might as well carry on... until after the weekend, holiday, birthday, or other event. And then, because we know we will be going without something soon, we binge on anything and everything we can, as there will soon be a famine going on in our body. It's worth mentioning here, that when our body feels it's in famine mode, it actually stores much more than normal. So, often by eating less and causing ourselves stress, we can feel fatter and slower because the body is trying to hold onto its reserves. When we fall into giving ourselves a hard time for being lazy, fat, or having no willpower, we actually reinforce those negative pathways in the brain, meaning that we not only slip into them easier each time, but that we also actually reinforce the messages the brain is giving to the body. This means that we keep ourselves looking exactly the way we do not wish to. Where our attention goes, energy flows!

So, instead of giving yourself a hard time, simply pick yourself back up, appreciate the wonderful and joyous time you had with your friends' take-away and prosecco, and grab a juice or the fermented food and simply carry on being kind, gentle, and loving to yourself in any way you can. You can choose to make healthier and ultimately happier choices for yourself again right there and then; not the next day, week or month, but right then. It doesn't have to be all or nothing. It doesn't have to be that you are on a strict diet or not. It can simply be that you enjoy your roll around with your fun friends, but now you can enjoy feeling good in your body with some healthier options.

And, remember what I said earlier... the fermented foods and drinks help you to process and detox from the 'naughty' foods, so have them side-by-side. When you have a bottle of wine, try to drink plenty of water to flush yourself through and keep hydrated. If you have pizza, then have a big-ass salad on the side of it, and if you have a sugary, wheaty cake then stick a big pile of berries on top.

It really doesn't have to be one thing or the other; you can enjoy your food and still enjoy the body you live in, too.

The frame of mind in which we eat has as much to do with our health and weight as the food we are actually eating!

When I was battling with food and body image, I would often eat good food but in a really bad frame of mind (hating it and the process of buying, preparing, and eating it), or I would binge eat (hating myself all the while and the food for making me fat). When we eat (and also exercise) in a bad frame of mind, we cause a stress response around not just eating, but food in general and even shopping for and preparing food. When our body is in a stress response, it does not absorb the nutrients from the food so well, which can cause IBS-type symptoms and food intolerances.

Have you ever noticed that when you eat 'naughty' food but do so in a good frame of mind, you don't feel so bad mentally or physically afterwards? Yet when you eat 'naughty' (or sometimes good) foods in a poor frame of mind, they do not affect you in the same way? It's the same with wine! If you drink a bottle of wine in a bad frame of mind, compared to in a good frame of mind, it affects you in a very different way, both while drinking it and the following day. Ha!

Becoming a conscious food shopper, preparer, and eater, allows you to be more mindful of your food choices, your feelings behind them, how amazing it is to have so many beautiful foods, and to eat in a grateful, nurturing, nourishing, and healthy way. Shovelling food in not only means that we eat past our full point, but we often eat foods we would prefer not to, don't chew our food enough (making the harder to process and digest), and then don't absorb and utilize as much as we could from the amazing foods we consume.

Being a conscious and kind food shopper, preparer, and eater, is one of the best things you can do for your health. Even if the foods aren't all that good for you, you will start to build a better relationship with what you are putting into your system, and how you feel about your body.

One of my favourite things to do is to find pretty unhealthy foods then create healthier versions of them.

I like cake! In fact, I LOVE cake! I do not wish to never eat cake again, or to feel bad every time I do, so I spend time playing around in the kitchen making healthy (yet super yummy – this bit is important) cakes. This means I can not only enjoy the cakes I eat, but I can even enjoy seconds, but at the same time I am actually nourishing my body with tons of lovely vitamins and minerals rather than with sugars, wheats, and colourings.

If you would like some ideas for healthy, yet super yummy cakes and other foods, then check out my blog here: *www.faithcanter.com/blog/*

Or my first two books here

www.faithcanter.com/books/

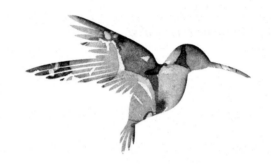

HEART WIDE OPEN

When we move from our head to our heart, we move from comparison, judgement, confusion, and fear, to compassion, kindness, clarity, and love. It's good to remind ourselves that when we are feeling these perceived negative feelings, it is simply a reminder that we have moved away from our hearts and back into our heads again.

As I mentioned earlier in this book, we came into this world heart-centered, but then learned that to fit into society we needed to be head-centered. So, what we do now is re-educate ourselves to live more in our hearts than our heads. When we are trying to fit in, we can feel alone, conflicted, and scared. And when we start to take those first steps to being ourselves – and not like anyone else – then we can still feel lonely, conflicted, and scared. But when we are ourselves, the more like-minded and beautiful people come into our lives and the less anything else matters. One beautiful way to not get caught up in the perceived negative feelings I have mentioned, is to realise that everything is love. Love is everywhere within you, in everything you come into contact with, and life itself.

I often ask my clients to play with being Heart Wide Open. By this I mean to walk around with your heart open. Feel an opening where your heart is, an expansion, an encapsulation of life, a connection to all. Feel it like you are viewing the world through an open heart. Try it now. If you are sitting on a bus, in your office, or in bed, just give it a go. Imagine your heart is opening up (much like a flower), you feel it filling your body, then the area around you, you feel the connection to all that is around you and beyond. You realise you are no longer alone, no longer isolated, because you are love and you see love all around. Love cannot be lonely, love is perfect, as are you and your life.

Recently, I was walking my dogs early in the morning and in a lot of pain from an injury I had sustained. The cold, icy weather was making it worse. I found myself slipping into negative thinking about having to get up early to walk the dogs by myself, in the icy weather, with wounded hands. After a few moments, though, I caught myself in this negative cycle and laughed out loud. 'Oh, you pesky mind of mine, you almost had me there!' When I realised I'd got stuck in my thoughts, and thus become closed off to all that was happening around me in this beautiful world, I flipped it. I literally moved my awareness from my head to my heart, and started to walk along with my heart wide open instead. I instantly felt more connected, less isolated, less pained and cold, and more open, grateful, and in love with the woods, the dogs, and my life again. Instantly!

I know this sounds super-simple, but it really is just that. Practising being heart wide open opens you up to life, to its opportunities and its beauty. And when we are not in battle with ourselves (within our head), we also have more energy and more motivation to enjoy life's adventures.

I recently posted a video about this on social media and one of my followers, who has been ill for a long time and who struggles with her energy at social gatherings, said she would try this concept that day. She was going out to a function and was worried it would drain her, as these events usually did. I told her to report back about her findings. She did, and she said she had found it much easier to deal with the gathering; not only that, she had even enjoyed it and managed to stay until the end.

You see, being heart wide open is a non-conflicted, non-stressed, non-draining space to hang out in. It's open, aligned, in flow, and in love with the world. This has a huge impact on us, as we have often become programmed to think negatively much of the time, especially about ourselves, our lives, and about others. This is not only draining, but it also triggers physical responses.

So, just for today, try being heart wide open. Just for now, in this moment, give it a go.

Set a reminder on your phone to go off two or three times a day, to remind you to be heart wide open. Set reminders to be heart wide open when you are walking to work, walking the dogs, or with friends or family (especially if you consider them to be draining).

When you stop fighting yourself and the world, the world does not drain you. In fact, it energises, fuels, and empowers you!

Whenever I am not feeling the love for myself, the person in front of me, or life, I know I have slipped into my head and then see it as an invitation to return to my heart. When we see perceived bad things simply as invitations to return to a

place of love, then the perceived bad things don't seem quite so bad.

Life wants us to be happy, it wants us to be love; it's we humans that think it wants something different from us. So, recognise the invitations from life to do just this, to return to the love of who you are and the life you have.

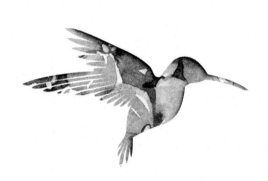

GETTING HORNY FOR LIFE

There are no ordinary moments.

Dan Millman,
Way of the Peaceful Warrior

The above is one of my all-time favourite quotes, from one of my favourite authors and my favourite book and film. This book completely changed my life. I went from feeling sorry, disgusted, and despairing of myself and my life, to seeing each moment in a very different way (even though I was still housebound with ME/CFS). There really are no ordinary moments. Life is a series of magical moments that we, through our conditioning, have learned not to notice and interact with. The good news, though, is that this can be easily be undone! How?

Become a celebrator!

Celebrate all that is beautiful in life, the birds, the flowers, the sun, the rain, the birthdays – oh, come on, what's the point in playing the 'I'm getting older game', really? Yes, we all are, so enjoy it rather than fight it! Celebrate the anniversaries, the cycle of life (birth and death), walks with your dog (or dogs in my case). Celebrate the road trips, the rail journeys, your job, your health, your eyes to see, your nose to smell, your ability to write, the beauty of every day as it unfolds. Nothing else has to change other than you throw those beauty blinkers off and celebrate all that makes up your life.

So many people don't get to live a full life for many reasons, and you may feel you aren't living a full life for your own reasons. I know I did. I was in the pits of despair about how crappy my life was. But you know, you can make a difference, you can break this habit of thinking and install a new, beautiful, and healthy one.

The more we practise being a celebrator rather than a destroyer, the more things in our life we find to celebrate. And don't we all really want a life we are celebrating rather than dishonouring? We have each been granted a small amount of precious time on this magical planet; let's make it count, let's celebrate all its beauty, all its good and bad, all its growth, all its changes. There's no point – and a lot of energy lost – fighting what we perceive is happening, when celebrating what is *actually* happening nurtures a love of self and love of life that fills you up each and every day. Being a celebrator allows more life into your life and more love into your heart.

Practise this today! Set a reminder/alarm each hour or couple of hours that says, 'Become a Celebrator' or 'Celebrate what just happened'. And as soon as it goes off, find one thing near to you or that has recently happened to you, to celebrate. And I mean *really* celebrate. Bring it into your heart, open your heart to its beauty, its magic, and allow life to fill you up.

Becoming a celebrator allows you to see the good in what we perceive as bad. I could never before believe that good comes out of so much bad in the world – but it does, time and time again.

One of the things I started doing when I started my recovery from ME/CFS was to read other recovery stories. Not just from ME/CFS, but from everything – from terminal cancer, the horrors of war, rapes, and even AIDS (yes, AIDS – check out some of these stories online). In these stories, people shared the awful things they had gone through, but also and more importantly they shared how they had resolved these things, grown, wakened up to life, a calling, an openness, a love, and a change. They didn't blame others, God or life, they celebrated where they were, how they had achieved it, and how they were now helping and inspiring others, or changing how society perceived or did something now. From the bad came a life of celebrations.

So, when you look around and think there is nothing to celebrate, know that this is just your mind playing games with you. Notice this thought, allow it (but don't become consumed by it) and honor the thought/feeling. But then, from your heart and not your head, look around with the beauty blinkers thrown off once more and celebrate that you are seeing life through those beautiful see-ers, hearing it through those magical hear-ers, and smelling it through that beautiful smell-er. Then notice what those see-ers, hear-ers and smell-ers see, hear, and smell, and celebrate those. Before you know it, the snowball effect of being a celebrator will be unstoppable.

What's annoying you right now? Can you reframe it? What I mean is, instead of being annoyed by the noise of the planes overhead, by the dog barking along the street, or next door's car alarm, can you instead use this as a trigger for happiness? Sometimes we need reminders to generate new habits, and it's the same with happiness and/or health habits. So, why not use the things that annoy you as habit reminders instead? That way they become good things rather than bad things. You can get your horn on for those things, rather than them trigger resentment, judgement and annoyance in you.

What's annoying you right now? And what is it you are trying to achieve right now? If you are trying to remember to drop into your heart more, then use your neighbour's dog barking as a reminder to do that. (I can guarantee that you are not in your heart if you are annoyed with the dog anyway, ha!) Each time you hear the dog bark, remember how amazing it is to have ears to hear this, and a home to hear it from, then see it as an invitation to drop into your heart. This way, the dog barking becomes a good thing rather than an annoying thing.

I often find myself smiling from head to toe whilst walking down the road, being in a traffic jam, travelling on the bus, or waiting in a queue. Why? Because I am living a life of celebration. I am celebrating being able to walk down the road, feeling the weather on my face, for the fact I have a car to be stuck in traffic with, for friends being friends on the bus, and for my ability to stand in a queue. Fighting life gets us nowhere but feeling exhausted, yet celebrating does the opposite. It fills us up with life and thus life's energy. It's like being plugged into a Universal energy resource. How freaking awesome is that?

Become a celebrator and change the way you view your life and the world!

Never let a day go by without celebrating the awesomeness of life. There's no point in fighting life, there's no point in hating life, or even just feeling that it is all the same. Open your eyes, your heart, and your soul, and embody its greatness in all you do, say, and are. Become that celebrator who encourages others to be that celebrator. Life is sooooo worth celebrating!

The miracle is not to walk on water. The miracle is to walk on the green earth, dwelling deeply in the present moment and feeling truly alive.

Thich Nhat Hanh

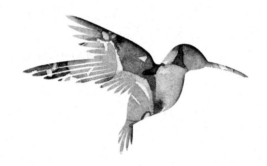

BECOMING A CREATOR

What has being creative got to do with loving yourself and your life more? Firstly, being creative is an expression of who we are, it's a way of expressing our emotions and some-times creating something beautiful, or at the very least creating something real. But that's not all. When we are creating, we are growing. And by creating, I don't mean just painting or drawing, I mean playing music, sewing, gardening, writing, tidying, working on a project, decorating, or a whole host of other things. I believe when we are not creating, growing, and moving forward, we slowly begin to die. We feel unfulfilled, unexpressed, unmotivated, and unheard. Actively taking time out to create a work of art or a new project fills us up.

We humans find it increasingly hard to stick to things that we feel we get very little from. I regularly see clients who can't stick to new diets, new exercise routines, relationships, careers, or other things in their life. Why? Because these things aren't fulfilling, they don't light them up, they aren't producing the results they want. However, it's easy to become a creator when the creating fills them up. So, how can you make your current creations more fulfilling? If they are things like art and garden-based creations, then you probably get fulfillment from the finished piece. However, when it's something like eating healthy, you may not be able to see the changes so easily and you get bored of salad, so it becomes harder to stick to it.

If the salad is boring, uninspired, and unfulfilling, then change it! I eat salad every day, but if it was just lettuce, tomatoes, and cucumber, I doubt I could face it, either! Create a salad that is beautiful, place it in an attractive bowl, and serve it with delicious accompaniments. Create a dinner that is fulfilling and beautiful for mind, body, and soul. You won't be eating from a lack/famine state, which will mean you are eating in a more nourishing and nurturing way for your body to utilise the goodness in your food.

Become a creator and create the food, situations, and life that you want. No-one wants to waste another year feeling stuck, unin-spired, and unfulfilled, so be the change. The only way things will change is if *you* change it. If your food isn't fulfilling, create food that is. If you are bored in your free time, create some projects that fill you up. And if your career or relationship isn't where you want it to be, stop focusing on all the crappy parts and start concentrating on creating happier parts.

If you want something different, you need to be the one to create it!

Stop focusing on what you don't have, and start creating the life you desire. Don't give your power/energy/attention to what you do *not* want, as that only reinforces those things. If, right now, you can't let go of what you don't want, try refocusing on it instead. What I mean by this is, rather than saying to yourself, 'I'm fat', say: 'I am currently embracing ways to become happier and healthier within my body.' This is not only a much kinder and softer way to communicate with yourself (and not causing you an underlying stress response), but you will start to reinforce this positive focus on your weight rather than the negative one of possibly 'being too fat'.

Only you can do this; no-one else can! Become the creator of your own destiny, stop wasting precious resources focusing on lack, and turn that energy to lustre instead!

Take some time now to schedule pleasure into your day, week, life. Consciously create the change you desire one calendar/diary entry or sticky-note at a time.

As you think certain thoughts, the brain produces chemicals that cause you to feel exactly the way you were thinking. Once you feel the way you think, you begin to think the way you think, the way you feel. This continuous cyclecreates a feedback loop called a 'state of being'.

Dr. Joe Dispenza

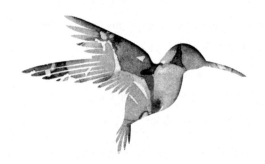

THE THOUGHTS ARE ONLY STORIES

There are no hopeless situations; there are only men who have grown hopeless about them.

Anonymous

We humans are amazing at feeling an emotion and then creating a back-story as to why we feel that emotion now. For example, I may wake up and feel instantly sad tomorrow morning (for no apparent reason). I will then go on a search – inside my own head – for the reasons why. My head will fire up in response and say, 'you feel sad because of X', and then a back-story is created to justify this and to reinforce this sad story. We could all be gold medallists at this, because we are totally awesome at it!

We are slaves to our suffering because we have learned this way of being. What if we could change this? What if we could unteach this belief and install a new one? What if we listened to our hearts and not our heads? You are not your stories. You are the sky, the birds, the trees, the leaves; you are the very nature of being.

The negative thoughts about yourself that you are currently listening and reacting to, are false. The false self that you have created through a story which you have made up or over-exaggerated to explain the feelings you are having. Have you noticed that those feelings came first and then the story unravelled in your head afterwards, not the other way around? Our thinking brain (which is where most of us hang out most of the time) creates stories about how we feel to justify these emotions, and these stories are based on our previous experiences, history, and habits. But when we bring our awareness away from the thinking brain and into the heart, we not only find clarity, inspiration, and truth, but we also come out of conflict and step into love.

So, when you realise that you have gone off into a story of why you feel the way you do, simply bring your awareness from the head to the heart. Rest in the space, place your hand on your heart, and breathe in and out of your heart. From this place, ask yourself: is this true? What nourishing and nurturing thing can I do for myself right now? And now stay there for as long as it takes to embrace being in your heart rather than in your head.

As you start to practise this, you may find that it can be many hours, days, or even weeks before you remember to do this, but the more you do it the easier and quicker it is to find your way back home to your heart each time. And eventually, you will only take a few moments – or hours at the most – before you have naturally slipped back into the heart space.

There is another beautiful way of realising we are stuck in our story of a feeling, and it was shared with me recently by the wonderful Abby Wynne (Hay House author, Energy Healer, Psychotherapist, and Shaman). Abby recommended that we write down our main stories – these are the ones that can be triggered in us often, and which we know well. There's usually 5 or 6 of them, but sometimes less, sometimes more. Abby suggests writing them all down, then when you realise you are in one of these stories, have a conversation with that story. This allows us to become an observer of the story/thoughts and not consumed by them, and helps us to realise that these stories are not us.

You could say things like: 'Hey, story of my unworthiness, thanks for stopping by, lovely to hear from you, but if you wouldn't mind popping off again, that would be grand.' Do you see how then the story is just that – a story; and not something we have to get involved with or be sucked under by? Love the story and let it go!

Another method I have been recently using myself and with my clients is called the 'Why Game'. Do you remember the game you used to play as a child, when someone (usually your parent or sibling) asked you to do something and you would respond with the question, why? And you would keep doing this until they or you had had enough. Well, if you suspect you are caught up in a story and you ask yourself 'why am I doing this?' and keep asking why, getting deeper and deeper to the core of what is happening, you will more often than not resolve being stuck in your story as you will realise what is actually behind it. So, if you are feeling crappy, ask yourself why, until you are under the story your mind has made up and have come to the raw emotion/feelings, and then keep asking why until you have no more why's to ask.

Doing at least one heart-centred meditation a day will help you to discover a new and easier way of being you, and will train your mind and body to slip into the heart more often and more easily than hanging out in the head.

I recently read a story by psychologist Dr. Dudley Calvert, about a man working on a railroad in Russia. He managed to get himself stuck in a refrigerator car and banged on the door and screamed for ages, but no-one heard him. Finally, he accepted he was going to die, and sat down to write a message on the wall with his fingers. 'I'm becoming colder now. Starting to shiver. Nothing to do but wait. I am slowly freezing to death. Half asleep now. I can hardly write. These may be my last words.' And they were. A few hours later, the man was found dead. The thing is that they found out later that the refrigeration unit on the car was actually broken, and there was enough air in there to last a very long time. The man had believed himself dead! He had believed his own mind so strongly that this had shut down his body.

What are you believing? What are you reinforcing? What could you love and let go of?

As a single footstep will not make a path on the earth, so a single thought will not make a pathway in the mind. To make a deep physical path, we walk again and again. To make a deep mental path, we must think over and over thekind of thoughts we wish to dominate our lives.

Henry David Thoreau

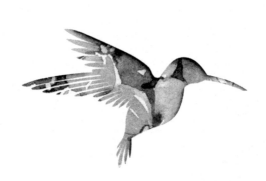

EMBRACING YOUR SHADOW SELF

t's easy to love the things we love about ourselves... well, easier!

I am sure, if we're all honest, we will find that we like at least a few things about our self – it might be our hair, our eyelashes, our nails, how we care about our friends, that we are good at maths, or that we care deeply about animals or the planet. So, this part is fairly easy, if we think about what we like.

What becomes trickier is embracing the side(s) of us that we don't like. That might be our judgements about our friend's hair or make-up, our own bum or belly, our lazy tendencies when no-one is looking, or even the fact that we actually don't like a family member or a friend very much at all. I am sure that, again with some thought, this list would be much longer than the other list. We have become pro's over the years at listing off all the things we dislike about ourselves. But true self-love comes from embracing our shadow side(s), the side(s) of us that we do not like. Trying to love our self when not loving *all* of our self, really doesn't work. You probably already know this, as you have no doubt tried. As I mentioned earlier in this book, acceptance is the key. The key to our happiness, our freedom, and our love of self, others, and even the world.

It was when I truly started accepting the parts of myself that I did not like so much – those shadow sides – that I finally found true peace with myself, my body, and my life.

Next time you feel yourself judging a part of you – for whatever reason – as soon as you catch yourself doing this, try telling yourself some of the following:

1. It's ok to feel this way, I'm human and I am having a human experience.

2. It's ok that I judged myself in this way.

3. I am not going to give myself a hard time for giving myself a hard time (that's the crazy brain getting crazier).

4. I am ok with this thought process, it makes me human.

5. It's ok that I judged myself.

6. I accept the thing I judged about myself, because judging it does not serve me or it.

7. I accept it that I am like this at this moment.

8. I know that when I rest in a place of acceptance of this part of me, I no longer fight it/me and reinforce it with my thinking.

9. I know that when I accept things as they are, the things I accept have the space to change if they need to.

10. I let go of fighting myself in this moment right now.

11. Just for today, I choose a different way.

When you rest in your heart, you will find there is no judgment there. Just love – pure love for you and for this part of you. Stay in this place for a long as possible, and play with sharing love with this part of you. See yourself and this judged part of you with a heart wide open. You know you are the divine, right? We all are! You are an embodiment of the divine, and in being so you are pure love; all parts of you are pure love.

The same goes for our past. The past has made us who we are now. But I have noticed what often happens is that we start to become ok with where we are now, but our past still bothers us. So much so that we will often try to distract ourselves from it. I know I did this. I didn't want to think about the perceived bad things I had done in my past – the drugs, drinking, men, lying, and cheating. Now was ok, I was in a good place that I loved, and I had started to love me. However, I wasn't embracing how I had come to be me. I wasn't embracing this big-ass shadow side from my past.

I started slowly working with my heart about my past. I drew a timeline of my life, year by year (and in certain parts of my life, month by month), and began plotting on to it all the parts of me I was still judging. It was quite a surprise to see it laid out in all its glory, but there it was. And from that, I noticed that after each perceived bad phase in my life, there had been a big shift. *Interesting*, I thought. I noted that every 'rock bottom' had in fact moved me closer to where I was now. I started to note, next to the items on the timeline, what I had learned from each one of them, or from each phase. I was surprised again how much there was. I even noted which new people had come into my life and what I had learned from them. Then I noted down things like how that perceived bad thing had pushed me to move to a new place, or to start a new career, or whatever else it had done.

The timeline started to take on a life of its own. I couldn't believe this was me – my life, my shadow history, all the things I had hated about my past. I just kept going and going until I ran out of steam. When I had stopped, I could clearly see that without each and every one of these perceived bad times, I wouldn't be the self that was now. I had needed these things to help me grow, to help me find other ways of living and being me, to help me understand and to help me change how I felt and how I was living.

You are not hurting because someone hurt you, but because you still have raw wounds that are being scratched/triggered. We hurt ourselves by not resolving old wounds; no-one does it to us. In fact, the hurt is really an invitation to resolve that trigger. It's, in fact, a good thing (don't shoot me!). And as a result, you can use this hurt as a way to embrace and resolve your shadow self and/ or your past.

When you learn to love hell, you will be in heaven.

Thaddeus Golas

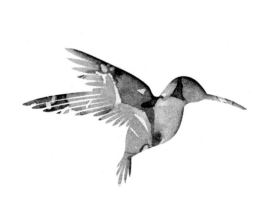

LETTING GO OF FEAR

So tired, so exhausted, so drained, so starved, starved of fun,
starved of energy, starved of conversation and inspiration.

Losing a little, a little bit more of myself every time I leave the house.

Going within, protecting what's left,

hurting more and more, being me less and less.

I hit rock bottom, again and again,

and finally I've had enough and I choose a different way.

I choose to heal, I choose to believe,

I choose to leave what I thought was, for what is.

A new journey begins, a new light is within.

It's far from easy, in fact it hurts.

I see a life when I let go of my comfort zone.

And I feel love where I once felt fear.

A life of no regret, a life that was meant to be.

A life of love, a life of totally and utterly being me!

When you are fearing your future, you are not living your moment!

Many people fear a relationship ending, losing their job, not having enough money, and death (theirs or other people's). What is the point in fearing the future? What is the point in fearing the unknown? It keeps us stuck, it keeps us closed off, and it keeps us from living fully. A loved one, or even your future self, would wish you to live your life fully, to trust, to embrace, and to love. If your 80-year-old self could tell you that all that worry, that fear, and that stress never created a roof over your head, never kept that relationship going, never stopped you or anyone else from dying, and that – you know what? – everything worked out just fine: would you listen? Would you live a little more now?

That thinking brain which plays the doubt game, will always doubt, will always hold you back, and will always keep you closed off to living life fully.

Firstly, play with the doubt, see if you are ok with it simply being there, hanging out. If not, then maybe, just maybe, it's here to teach you something – perhaps another message from the body to sort your 'stuff' out? Listen to what it's telling you, be open to its words, and then embark on a process of resolution and invite more love into your once fearful heart.

Life was a scary place for me. I was fearful of losing my hubby, the dogs, family, my health worsening and bad things happening left, right, and centre. The world was not a safe place to me. But my thoughts about the world were exactly what was making the world so bad to me. It caused me so much stress and anxiety every day, thinking about what could go wrong, that my health was getting worse and worse, and my life smaller and smaller.

What I learned to do instead was to start to make friends with these feelings. Allowing them and my anxiety to be there, to not fight them any longer, and to just embrace their being. Once I did that, I started to play with the idea of trusting life and my journey through it. I or a family member might pass away tomorrow or it may be 30 years from now, but worrying about it would only cause me a great deal of stress, and hinder my health.

So, I started to trust in life's journey. When the fear would rise up in me, I would feel it, allow it, love my humanness, and see it as an invitation to embody a little more trust in this magical journey. As I have mentioned before, life is happening *for* us, not against us, and when we see this we can pass through the fear more quickly and rest in the love of life, its redirections, and its magic with more ease.

Learning to trust has been one of my biggest hurdles and one of my greatest lessons. When you have spent a lifetime not trusting yourself or anyone around you – especially if you have been hurt time and time again – it feels quite alien to trust in yourself and in others again. It almost feels wrong on some level, but only because you have a lifetime's habit of not trusting, with a lifetime of reasons and beliefs why that is a perfectly logical way to be. It's protected you, right? It's been your defence mechanism. And if you don't trust, then you don't get let down, because you never expect anything much from anyone anyway. Wrong! The only thing it's protecting you from is living a full and happy life.

If you struggle to embrace trust, then drop down into the heart, rest your awareness there, place your hand there, and breathe in and out of there. Now, from this place, ask yourself: is this fear true? And then ask yourself, what would love do?

I love this question: what would love do? It moves us instantly from fear to love, and if we are fully in our hearts before asking it, it allows us to hear our heart's highest hope for us in this moment.

Letting go allows flow!

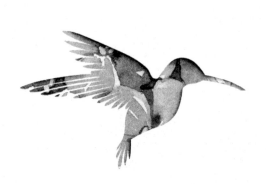

FINDING PURPOSE IN FLOW

When I am totally in flow, I have more energy and inspiration than I know what to do with. When I am not, I do not. It's really that simple!

really dislike this thing in entrepreneurial circles where they say: 'Find someone doing what you want to be doing and copy them.' I want to scream Nooooooooooooo whenever I hear this. Be you, be you in all your beauty, with all your perceived flaws, all your rawness, all your perceived mistakes, all that makes you gloriously you. Just be you! Do what feels right, what your gut/body/mind/ soul is telling you feels right. Remember she/he speaks to you; whispers your soul's desires, your comforts, loves, and purposes.

When you copy someone else, you are not being true to who you are, you give your power away, you do not listen to what your body and mind is trying to tell you. When you are listening, when you are living in that place of flow, that place of alignment, that place of being unconflicted, then *that's* the very place where people will find you, events will happen; job offers, relationships, and moves will all occur for your greater good. This place of listening, this place of non-conflict, is where you will feel truly inspired and empowered, and where you will inspire and empower others.

Going off searching for your purpose is you being in a place of conflict with where you are now. It's unlikely you will find your purpose from a place of conflict, a place of not being in flow, aligned, and inspired. When you are in this place of conflict, you are stuck in the thinking brain, trying to change where you are now. The thinking brain will only try to think its way towards dozens of potential 'purposes' and many never quite hit the mark. The thinking brain isn't where our purpose in life comes from; as you may have already guessed, it comes from the heart!

The thinking brain will get its chance to join the purpose party later on down the line, when you need to organize yourself to do things in line with your purpose.

Instead of going off searching for your purpose, just embrace 'being present', 'listening' and 'resolving' instead. As we resolve the conflicts and imbalances that our body is telling us about, and learn to listen to and love ourselves and our lives more, our purpose floods through, backed up by our passion, energy, and joy. Finding your purpose shouldn't be a chore, an upset or a conflict, it should come naturally through the nurturing and nourishment of who you are.

Embrace the not-knowing, concentrate on being more of what you came here to be. By resolving conflict, experiencing life fully, and living with a heart wide open, you will see and feel more of life's opportunities, guidance, and redirections happening in front of you. From that place of openness, you will find your purpose –

not from the closed-off place of the thinking brain, of the trying-to-fix, change, or improve place. So, spend more time listening to your body, spend more time in meditation, spend more time in awareness, and spend more time accepting the beauty of everything that makes you *you*. There you will find your true purpose and there you will find your joy!

Unbury yourself,

let a little life in,

shake a little dirt off,

see a little more light,

nurture yourself,

nourish yourself,

feed and water yourself,

feed your soul.

In doing so, you grow,

In doing so, you flow,

In doing so, you'll see,

the true purpose of you!

When living in your true seat of power, your true seat of inspiration, and following what brings you joy, you will know instantly when someone or something hinders this for you. Your energy will most likely dip, your inspiration may slide, and things start to feel forced and not flowing, as the thinking brain takes over.

Be aware of this change – it's just an invitation to listen to the body and mind again. Notice when your energy has dipped or when the thinking brain is trying to produce something creative for you – which it can't do very well, and which may make you feel you can't do it very well. But you can; it's just head and heart have become switched. Be aware of this change within you, learn to feel it early on, and learn to see it as an invitation to return to your heart. Ask your heart: what would love do? The heart only has your best interests at 'heart', whereas the head is ego and story-based. The head won't fix your writer's block, it won't give you more energy to get more done; it will likely drain you, consume you, and make you feel like you are not good enough for this purpose of yours. Bring yourself back into the heart space, your creative place, your inspiration place, and your flow place.

I have lost count of the times I've suddenly found myself drained and unable to create whatever it is I am trying to create, or that I have no time for some TLC. I then find myself some 'heart' time, and find that not only do I feel more energized from this time, but I am then more inspired and more creative. And even though I have less time (because I have taken this 'heart' time), I still manage to get so much more done. If you feel you have no time for you, then this is exactly the time to hang out in your heart, because you'll feel more energized, aligned, flowing, and inspired afterwards. And what you create will be all the better for it, as it will be created from the heart instead of from the head.

Being you will see you through!

Anything else may exhaust you, maybe make you ill, and likely make you feel unsatisfied. You will struggle to be you from the thinking brain, because the ego gets in the way. Practise being in your heart centre whenever you can, and realise your true potential, power, and purpose, and your true love of yourself and your life. If you are bored, overwhelmed, or exhausted, you have become disengaged from your heart – so re-engage, rejuvenate, and restore your heart compass, and she'll get you back on course.

You will find a powerhouse of energy when working from your heart rather than your head. You will shine with true authenticity, and others will notice and be attracted to this. Be you and only you, and you will shine with purpose, and your purpose will bring with it abundance in many areas of your life.

When you live a life of love, there is never a feeling of lack. And when there is no feeling of lack, and you are doing all you can to invite more love in, then your purpose will always provide for you and your life.

Next step, follow your fun! Your fun, those things that light you up, which feel light (and not heavy) and make your heart sing, those things are for you, those things can flow into purpose, those things will open you up, so you can see and feel your purpose more clearly.

Follow your fun!

What you love is a sign from your higher self of what you are here to do.

Sanaya Royan

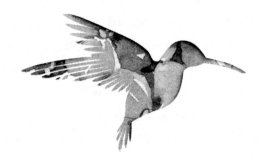

GETTING NAKED!

S cared of having fun? What's that all about? Scared because of what we'll look like, of what people will think, of illness, of beliefs and programming, scared of rejection, not feeling enough, not being worthy? Scared for the sake of being scared? Oh, and then the moment is gone and the choice is made, then we missed it, again!

Those things you think disempower you are actually here to empower you! The only real way to pass through a difficult time without it imprinting on you is to see the expansion of your own evolution within it.

I have evolved beyond my wildest dreams with each of the perceived crappy things that has happen to me in my life. From abuse, drug use, and various illnesses, to ME/CFS and a whole heap of other things. If it wasn't for these potential disempowering episodes in my life, I wouldn't be here writing to you and having the privilege to assist others with their journey. I lead a life much fuller than I ever thought possible, and I know with each hurdle that I come across I will continue to evolve; I have 100% success rate with it... I am still here, after all!

You do, too! You have a 100% rate of getting through everything in your life, because you are here, right here, right now!

The perceived crappy things are fuel for a fuller, happier, and healthier life. We just need to learn ways to harness the power of these situations rather than allow ourselves to be disempowered by them. I use such situations to fuel my empowerment in the following ways...

1. I remember I have a 100% success rate of being ok!

2. I trust that the expansion of my own evolution will come when I stop fighting the situation, myself, and others.

3. I remember that fighting the situation drains my energy and resources, as I really am only fighting myself.

4. I look for the lessons/gifts in the situation. I actively search out how this will allow me to grow and what I can do to harness this.

5. I remind myself that sometimes I have to let go to grow. Holding onto old habits, people, thoughts, memories, situations, grievances, and belongings, does little for our growth and actually keeps us stuck. Letting go can be a fundamental part of growth, even when it hurts like a bitch! ;0)

6. I remind myself that the stress and anxiety I feel is all created within me, it's my own inner reaction to a situation. I have the ability to react differently and in a way that impacts my own health and wellness positively rather than negatively.

7. I repeatedly ask myself this question: what would love do? This neutralises almost any situation where I feel doubt, resentment, judgment or hurt. If you are being unkind to yourself or to others, this one question will bring you out of that thought process and into a more heart-centred place of

nurturing yourself and/or the situation or person(s) troubling you.

8. Bad things aren't happening to me because I am a bad person (even though this is what I thought for much of my life). Perceived bad things are happening to me because I need a shift in my life, a redirection. Simply surviving is not acceptable to me. I want to live fully and completely, and to do this you sometimes need a big-arse wake-up call. Otherwise, one day easily fades into another and another, and before you know it, another year has gone by with nothing much changing.

9. I celebrate the good things happening around me; every single one of them.

10. I spend time hanging out in my heart, spending my time with my heart wide open. Things look and feel very differently then, even though mostly nothing has changed on the outside.

11. I value my place in the world! Every night, I list ways in which I have added value to the world, in any tiny way.

12. I remind myself that I am a walking, talking miracle, moving around on a magical ball of gas, water, and air, in an infinite Universe.

13. I listen to myself and the messages I am being given to resolve things I have been triggered to feel.

14. I feel those pesky feelings, each and every one of them.

15. I learn to communicate better with myself and others around me. I listen more, I'm kinder, more committed, and more open!

16. I remind myself: This Too Shall Pass! And when I do all the above, it does pass!

The more I practise the above, the easier it comes each time. I find myself spending less and less time in thought processes that disempower me, and more and more time in places of actively seeking out how these can empower me instead. Even this thought process by itself is empowering. Actively seeking ways in which something can empower you instantly allows less of your power to be lost to the situation. This, in turn, allows you more clarity and openness to see your way through it.

Being someone who can easily slip into a depressive nature, I have found it incredibly easy for me to drop into the pits of despair at the slightest little thing over the years. I thought the world, my body, and the people around me, were all against me. I see now, though, that it was only ever my own mind I was fighting. It has been like a revolution for my soul to realise this. A revolution for the expansion of my evolution! How totally awesome is that? ;0)

I have found that the more I let go of trying to conform, of judging others, of not being enough, and of trying to be anything else but me, then the happier and healthier I am and the happier and health-ier people around me are, too. I call this getting naked, embodying, and exposing what makes me *me* on every level. The more I do this, the less I am bothered by other people's views, and the less I see the ugliness which I used to see that I felt made me *me*.

The more *you* you are, the happier you will be!

The more you let go of the mask, the covers, the fake you that you think people want to see and be with, the more genuine and lovely people you will attract into your life. Why? Because they will be attracted to your authenticity, you will shine brightly and beautifully, being brilliantly you, you and no-one else!

It's time to get spiritually naked, let go of the pretence, let go of the lack, of the not enough, and of the need to be anyone but you. Bask in your own beauty, of life's beauty, and know that we all came here to love, to be love, and to share love. Nothing else matters, nothing!

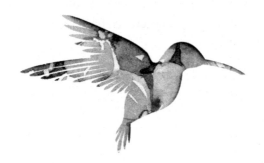

CHOOSE LOVE

Walking. I am listening to a deeper way. Suddenly all my ancestors are behind me. Be still, they say. Watch and listen. You are the result of the love of thousands.

Linda Hogan

What would love do?

I have asked myself this question many, many times. The question helped me move on from my marriage, to love myself more, listen to my body, and write this book. It's a powerful question and I urge you to try using it yourself.

I have lived and breathed every word of this book. I honestly never thought I would be happy, never thought I would grow to love my body and my being, and I never thought things could be different. But one day – much like at the turning point with my ME/CFS – I decided enough was enough and that I was not prepared to continue my life like this any more. There had to be another way, and I was going to find it!

I have tried many techniques, many ways of not being me some more, many ways of not embodying all that makes me *me*. Changing who I was some more, trying to 'fix' myself, hating the process, causing more stress, and feeling less alive. Until I started to practise what is on the pages of this book. These pages, these words, and these thoughts, saved me from getting sucked under by my perceived crappiness! The bad feelings come still, but I welcome their existence, their messages, and their gifts, and I allow myself to feel them without getting caught up in the story and sucked under once more.

But most of all, the one thing I can share with you, is that if you keep choosing love, over and over again, then there will be more love in your life, there will be less fear, there will be more ease, more life, and more flow. Keep making the choice of love, keep letting go of what's getting in its way, and keep allowing yourself to grow, allowing the redirections, and keep being totally and utterly you.

Consciously create the change in your life that you desire, but not from a place of conflict, not from a place of fear, and not from a place of not feeling good enough. Anything you do because you are not happy with where you are, will likely cause conflict within you. This, in turn, can cause a stress response around the choices you are making. Try to ensure your choices come from love, from your heart, and thus for your greater good, and without a background feeling of not being good enough or trying to prove yourself. The choice of love is the greatest choice you can make for yourself. So, just for now, just for today, choose love!

When you keep choosing love, loving yourself inside becomes easier because you give up fighting yourself and life.

And remember to consciously create the change you desire.

The words/learnings I share in this book are anchors of a new way of being, living, loving and letting go. Embody them fully, re-read the Consciously Creating Change chapter, and/or get to work scheduling in all those beautiful things you are going to do for yourself moving forward.

Follow your lightness, follow your loves, follow your fun, design the life you desire from a place of love and nurturing, and not from a place of lack. You are enough, you are in fact *more* than enough, because you are a human embodiment of divine love. There is no more enough than that!

It is our choices that show what we truly are, far more than our abilities.

Albus Dumbledore

BOOKS THAT ROCK MY WORLD!

Way of the Peaceful Warrior – Dan Millman

The Alchemist – Paulo Coelho

The Pilgrimage – Paulo Coelho

Body Calm – Sandy Newbigging

It's the Thought that Counts – David Hamilton

How the Mind Can Heal the Body – David Hamilton

How to Be Well – Abby Wynne

Awareness – Anthony De Mello

The Way to Love – Anthony De Mello

The Four Agreements – Don Miguel Ruiz

The Choice for Love – Barbara De Angelis

Mutant Message Down Under – Mario Morgan

Life's Golden Ticket – Brendan Burchard

A Simple Act of Gratitude – John Kralik

Taking the Leap – Pema Chodron

Lucid Living – Tim Freke

I Can See Clearly Now – Wayne Dyer

Longevity Now – David Wolfe

The Top Ten Things Dead People Want to Tell You – Mike Dooley

Last Child in the Woods – Richard Louv

Earthing: The Most Important Health Discovery Ever – Clinton Ober, Stephen Sinatra, and Martin Zucker

I am forever updating my favourite reading list and also my favourite inspiring films and documentaries list. For an up-to-date version of both, check out my blog posts below:

Inspiring Reads: www.*faithcanter.com/inspiring-reads/*

Inspiring Films & Documentaries

www.faithcanter.com/my-top-inspiring-documentaries-films/

Remember: what we are watching and reading regularly, forms part of what we are fueling our bodies, minds, and lives on, so choose wisely, choose happy, and choose inspiring wherever you can!

Lightning Source UK Ltd.
Milton Keynes UK
UKOW06f0952181017
311194UK00013B/896/P